THE SPIRIT OF
ANIMAL HEALING

ALSO BY DR. MARTY GOLDSTEIN

The Nature of Animal Healing

THE SPIRIT OF ANIMAL HEALING

An Integrative Medicine Guide to a Higher State of Well-being

DR. MARTY GOLDSTEIN

Illustrated by Emma and Ayla Goldstein

ST. MARTIN'S
ESSENTIALS
NEW YORK

First published in the United States by St. Martin's Essentials, an
imprint of St. Martin's Publishing Group

THE SPIRIT OF ANIMAL HEALING. Copyright © 2021 by Martin
Goldstein. All rights reserved. Printed in the United States of America.
For information, address St. Martin's Publishing Group, 120 Broadway,
New York, NY 10271.

www.stmartins.com

Designed by Steven Seighman

The Library of Congress Cataloging-in-Publication Data
is available upon request.

ISBN 978-1-250-24969-2 (trade paperback)
ISBN 978-1-250-24970-8 (ebook)

Our books may be purchased in bulk for promotional, educational, or
business use. Please contact your local bookseller or the Macmillan
Corporate and Premium Sales Department at 1-800-221-7945, extension
5442, or by email at MacmillanSpecialMarkets@macmillan.com.

First Edition: 2021

10 9 8 7 6 5 4 3 2 1

To my incredible wife, Meg.
Without her support, a book such as this
could never have been written.
And to my three beautiful daughters, Emma, Hana, and Ayla.
This beautiful family and their love for and interaction
with the animal kingdom tells me every day that the
path I chose is the right one.

To Ruth and Irv, aka Mom and Dad.
Thanks for having me as your son, and for your guidance when
I was growing up.
And your love for the animals you brought into our home,
so I could be who I am.

CONTENTS

INTRODUCTION

What's New?

Never doubt that a small group of thoughtful, committed citizens can change the world. Indeed, it is the only thing that ever has.
—MARGARET MEAD

In 1999, more than two decades ago, I published my first book: *The Nature of Animal Healing*. This revolutionary act challenged the existing veterinary establishment, which had trained and certified me, while introducing many thousands of pet parents to the principles of *integrative medicine*—the merging of traditional and alternative treatments into holistic medical practice. I helped pioneer integrative veterinary medicine, over the years gathering with me an ever-larger group of like-minded veterinarians and other animal experts. It was a lonely place to be in the beginning, but today I can proudly say that this emerging field we built together has improved the lives of millions of dogs and cats—in many cases extending their lives or saving them outright.

In the intervening years quite a few books have been published providing people with advice and recommendations for enabling nature to do what it does best—to naturally support the health of companion animals. As you'll learn as you read on, I firmly believe that it's not the primary job of veterinarians (or of any other doctors) to treat sick patients— it's to help them remain healthy in the first place.

We have done so many bad things to our environment, to the food we feed our animal companions, and to the dogs and cats who share their lives with us that illness is not the exception that it was millennia ago. Now it's expected—it's par for the course. We expect the dogs and cats in our care to get sick, and they do. Then we load them up with more vaccines than they need, more drugs than they need, more medical procedures than they need. As a result, they're sicker than ever.

This book is all about getting off the merry-go-round of traditional veterinary practice and trying something different. Something better. Something more natural. Something that offers the dogs and cats in your life the best opportunity to be healthy throughout *their* lives—and *ours*.

This book is *not* a do-it-yourself, how-to of integrative veterinary practice. You won't find twenty-five different recipes for the best home-cooked dog or cat dinners, and you won't find recommendations for specific brands of dog and cat food or supplements.

Why not?

First, if I've learned anything in my more than forty-five years of veterinary practice, it's that each dog, each cat is an *individual*. Like snowflakes, no two are alike. What's good for one dog might not be so good for another—even of the same breed or litter. For example, while I recommend the feeding of raw food, I've seen dogs and cats that simply don't do well on it—they end up with gastrointestinal upsets or other issues. That's why, throughout this book, I impress upon you the need to find the best integrative veterinarian you can, then allow that doctor to get to know your animal companions well. This is how you can be assured they will get the best care possible, perfectly tailored to their unique physiology and needs.

As Hippocrates said about the nature of human medicine thousands of years ago, "It is far more important to know what person the disease has than what disease the person has." These wise words also apply to our animal friends.

Second, as we all know, the world is changing faster than ever. This is as true in veterinary practice as it is in every other aspect of our lives. I can pretty much guarantee, for example, that any recommendation I might make for a specific brand of food or course of supplements would be out-of-date a year, five years, or a decade from now. New products and new therapies are introduced all the time, and old ones are discarded.

Consider that smartphones have only been with us for little more than a decade. What kinds of new things will those phones be able to do for us a decade from today? Just look at all the changes they've already been through. While I have no idea what new things my phone will be able to do ten years from now, I do definitely know that they will be quite different from anything any of us might imagine in our wildest dreams. Change is a given, and it's my goal for this book to remain as accurate and relevant as it can be for as long as possible.

Above all, my aim in writing this book is to provide you with a trusted source for the latest thinking in integrative veterinary practice. Some of it might seem to be out on the edge, but most everything we do today in integrative veterinary practice was *way* out on the edge back in the early seventies when I graduated from veterinary school. My advice to you, the reader and animal lover, is to open your mind to all the possibilities in the world and universe in which we live. We humans don't know everything there is to know—not by a long shot—and there is much still to learn. Most every day I learn something new about how to make the lives of dogs and cats and other animals (ask me about my flock of chickens!) better.

And we do love our animal companions. According to American Pet Products Association (APPA) statistics, Americans share their homes with some 90 million dogs and 94 million cats.[1] Not only that, but we spend more than $75 billion a year on *all* our animal companions (not just dogs and cats) for food, veterinary care, over-the-counter medications, grooming, and more.[2] For many of us, our animal companions are true members of our families whom we depend on for companionship, loyalty, and love. It's an inseparable bond that has been forged over millennia.

Thanks for joining me on my adventure to good health! Now, let's get started.

THE SPIRIT OF ANIMAL HEALING

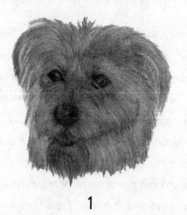

1

HOW FAR HAVE WE COME?

The microbe is nothing; the terrain is everything.
—LOUIS PASTEUR (ON HIS DEATHBED)

I graduated from the Cornell University College of Veterinary Medicine in 1973. In 2018, I returned to my alma mater to give a talk on integrative veterinary medicine. It was a homecoming of sorts, to a school that remains a bastion of conventional veterinary philosophy—just like almost all other university veterinary programs.

When I graduated, almost every veterinarian adhered strictly to the time-honored conventional practices taught by schools of veterinary medicine and the powers that be that subsidized these schools. The treatments were cut-and-dried. If an older dog had cancer, which was relatively rare at the time, you cut out the tumor, or you used powerful drugs to try to kill the cancerous cells—taking healthy cells along with them. If a cat had an infection or allergies, you gave it antibiotics, steroids, or other drugs. Sometimes these treatments had serious side effects, which could turn out to be worse than the original condition we were trying to fix. But we did it because that was what we were taught to do. Unfortunately, not much has changed today except that the number of treatments currently available has skyrocketed.

Cornell gave me one hour to speak and conduct a Q and A, and once word got out about my appearance, we filled the hall with eager students. You can't teach everything you need to know about integrative veterinary medicine in just one hour, so my major goal was to provide clear and compelling evidence of the efficacy of alternative treatments—that they *do* work.

While the school's old guard faculty and administration are still lukewarm to alternative therapies, the students are extremely curious about them and want to know more. I was told that when Cornell's administration surveyed the student body of the vet school a number of years ago, asking them if they had an interest in or affinity for alternative therapies, 93 percent said yes. But the board of trustees decided to ignore the results, explaining that if they ratified the survey and made changes to the curriculum, it would be like "letting the inmates run the prison and we can't set that precedent."

My presentation to the Cornell students wasn't about proving the school or its administration or professors wrong—it was about expanding the consciousness of the audience members, most of whom were students. Integrative veterinary medicine is the future of our profession, not a passing fad. Why? Because it works with mechanisms nature has created to heal instead of just treating symptoms.

Unfortunately, so much of conventional medicine suppresses these existing flows.

There's more to healing our animal companions than just diagnosing conditions, cutting out tumors, administering medications, or setting broken bones. A spiritual component is just as important, if not more important in many cases, and alternative and integrative therapies draw from this deep well.

Early in my presentations, I often project a slide about a book I received in 1981 as part of a select group of people, including Mrs. Anwar Sadat. The book, *The Hall of Records*, is about the human race finding the entombment of knowledge that was in existence during the time of the building of the Great Pyramid. It presents structural measurements, statistics, and levels of construction accuracy that are impossible to fathom knowing that the human race at that time had none of today's remarkable technology. According to just one passage from the book, "In more modern terms, the Pyramid contains enough material to build thirty Empire State Buildings."[1] Clearly, some level of knowledge and ability existed thousands of years ago that is well beyond our current comprehension.

And guess what? Acupuncture was laid down in about the same era. I showed my audience a human acupuncture model that has 361 discrete points covering its entire surface. I said, "Do you realize that back then they knew every single point and every single connection to a meridian of energy flow, and every connection to every internal organ at a time when it was sacrilegious to dissect the human body? And we're just now beginning to understand the workings of the more than 360 points and the meridians they are on that these ancient healers discovered thousands of years ago."

How did they know that?

Welcome to the future. Actually, "Welcome to the past" is exactly what I said to them.

Integrative medicine is both old and new, simultaneously. We know of plants and herbs that have been used by humans for thousands of years to address a variety of illnesses, and they could have an equal or better, more pronounced effect than do modern-day drugs. Many of these same plants and herbs can have a positive effect on the health and wellness of our animal companions.

For example, a study conducted by the University of Pennsylvania medical school revealed that the turkey tail medicinal mushroom has great success in treating one of the most nonresponsive cancers in dogs: hemangiosarcoma of the spleen.[2] According to the report, dogs with this cancer have a median survival time of eighty-six days, and chemotherapy doesn't hugely increase survival. While dogs typically live only three to six months when treated conventionally, they'll often live for more than a year when treated with this mushroom. Although the report doesn't discuss quality of life, I have used this medicinal mushroom and several others in clinical practice for more than fifteen years and have never seen any adverse reactions, especially compared to those of chemotherapy.

How can results such as these be explained—what does science have to say about this? Nature determines how we interact with the world around us—what harms us, what has a neutral effect, and what makes us stronger. My definition of science in the field of medicine is simply man trying to figure out what nature has already created.

I explained to the students what cancer is in simple terms, and how today we're looking for what cancer is out in the environment. Surprisingly, it doesn't exist out there. Simply put, cancer is caused by normal cells that go haywire because the immune system is no longer functioning properly. In the early days of a mammalian embryo's development, this organism is composed of numerous cells that are all exactly the same. Soon, however, the embryo goes through a miracle of nature called cell differentiation, in which different cell types begin to emerge and organize to form organs and structures in the developing fetus.

Again, simply speaking, cancer happens when something screws up this natural mechanism of cell differentiation. So, if we want to look for the cause of cancer in our animal companions and find the "cure," we have to look at those things that have fouled up natural development and normal cellular repair and replacement in their bodies. There are three key factors:

- Genetics
- Vaccinations
- Food

I reminded the audience that I was not there to cause controversy—I was there for each of them to learn and take away something new. When it comes to vaccinating animals, for example, I told them, "I am not anti-vaccination. I am pro-sanity. I feel that through the practice of standard vaccination protocols, we're actually violating our Hippocratic oath as doctors to do no harm." I then presented statistical evidence that a number of vaccines don't need to be given to dogs and cats every three years—as common veterinary practice today prescribes—and definitely not every year.

Unbeknownst to many veterinarians, standard vaccine potencies can be up to ten times what a Great Dane needs—imagine the effect of such a powerful substance on a much-smaller dog receiving the same exact dose. And many veterinarians continue to vaccinate sick animals when, on the package insert of every vaccine, it clearly states that the product is intended for use in healthy animals only. I suggested that Cornell should conduct scientific studies on the efficacy of vaccines and their adverse sequelae—and especially on the dose-to-weight relationship.

In 1978, my license to practice was verbally threatened for my treating of arthritic dogs with glucosamine sulfate. Now, supplement producers sell many millions of dollars' worth of glucosamine-type supplements every year, and no one's license is being threatened for recommending it. And guess who conducted the groundbreaking study demonstrating that CBD oil is effective for pain relief in arthritic dogs? Ironically, it was a team of researchers led by Associate Professor Joseph Wakshlag at Cornell University, and the study was published just a few months before my presentation. As I told the attendees in the auditorium, "It's time for you to listen."

Many of the students who attended my presentation were floored—they loved it. My hope is that they will really listen—and then act by bringing their desire to learn this emerging information to the faculty, administration, and board of trustees. The health, happiness, and well-being of many thousands of dogs and cats will soon be in their hands.

MY SWISS VISION

Years ago, soon after I joined my brother's veterinary practice in Yorktown Heights, New York, and then became a partner, one of my clients was Edgar Bronfman Sr. Edgar's family made its fortune primarily through their alcohol-distilling company, Seagram, and Edgar served for a time as chairman of the company.

Edgar's son Matthew, who was living in Washington, D.C., had a young Labrador named Taylor, after Taylor Vineyards, which was one of the family's wine companies. The dog had a degenerative, heredity shoulder condition called osteochondritis dissecans, and the known effective treatment at the time was surgical repair. It was like hip dysplasia, which was a common degenerative condition of the hips in those days—especially with German shepherds.

Edgar had Taylor flown to New York for a consultation. I examined the dog and put him on a regimen of supplements. A few months later, I got a call from Matthew. He told me that a new X-ray of Taylor's shoulder showed it was back to normal—100 percent.

"What are you doing?" he asked me.

"You know, I'm starting to get into alternative medicine."

"No, no, no. What are you doing? Can I come up and visit you?"

"Absolutely."

During Matthew's visit, we talked about the holistic-pet-care company I was starting with my family, and Matthew told me he was interested in investing in it. The first investment of $30,000 from the Bronfman family helped start the family-based company called Lick Your Chops. The first store was built, then several others followed.

When Matthew Bronfman married his first wife, Fiona, he flew me to Gstaad, Switzerland, for the wedding, all expenses paid. We were in the Swiss Alps overlooking a beautiful mountain valley.

One morning, after days of partying, I decided to go for a run—I desperately needed to get some oxygen inside me to clear my head. I turned on my Sony Walkman and ran up a beautiful Alpine mountain road near where we were staying. All of a sudden, two little dogs came flying down a driveway at me, barking viciously. I stopped in my tracks and looked directly at them.

My mind was still a little fuzzy, but in a serious tone I asked the dogs, "Excuse me? Do you know who you are barking at?" They froze. "You're barking at the person who is someday going to save your entire kingdom. So, if I were you, I would just stop and go back to your house."

Although I was just kidding around, to my amazement the two dogs put their tails between their legs and slowly sauntered up the driveway back to the house.

As crazy as this may sound, that's the vision I had that revealed to me the person I was about to become. My purpose in life was to save the lives of animals—as many as I possibly could during my life. I didn't know that it was going to take me forty-five or fifty years to get there, but it did.

As I was going through life building my veterinary practice, things got tough. My brother and I sold our old practice when Bronfman agreed to invest because we were going to create this huge business with Lick Your Chops. But the funding didn't come through in time—we were deeply indebted, debt beyond what you can imagine. My brother set up a small veterinary practice and started to see animals in his garage just to make ends meet because he had a family of four to support. It became so popular that he rented space at a kennel, which became the current Smith Ridge Veterinary Center (which was located on Smith Ridge Road in Salem, New York).

Being single, I was doing relief work. I was so broke, I would get up Monday morning at 4:30 a.m., cook eight ears of corn, brown rice, and lettuce, then go to my first job all day Monday and the ER Monday night. I would drive two hours up to my friend Howard's practice outside Woodstock and work all day Tuesday. I drove down to Queens Boulevard and worked the ER in Queens, where my life was always at risk, all Tuesday night. Then Wednesday I would work at my brother's clinic. I would work those three days in a row, maybe getting four to six hours of sleep in three days if I was lucky, and I would make enough money to pay all my bills *and* buy gas, corn, brown rice, and lettuce. That's how my life was, and that's when my Swiss vision really kicked in—over and over—keeping me going through those difficult times.

Then finally, when funding came in, my brother's expenses

were covered. He sold Smith Ridge Veterinary Center to me and I took it over in 1984. But life just kept getting tougher and tougher for me. I was working extremely hard, and every time I took on a new case and treated the animal with non-traditional means, I felt I was putting my license at risk. Because of that, I wasn't able to charge as much for my services as regular veterinarians were charging for accepted, conventional treatments. Pursuing a career in conventional veterinary medicine would have made things easy for me. Give a shot of cortisone and annual vaccines, remove a tumor, or put a dog or cat on antibiotics to provide some temporary relief.

I was constantly tempted to give up my integrative veterinary practice, to take the easy way out. But every time I decided that it was finally time to give it up, I would go back to the vision I had had in Gstaad and say to myself, "That vision was real and if you give up, that vision becomes not real, so you can't give up." That vision kept me going through decades of hell until I came out the other side.

THE NEW PRINCIPLES OF SPIRITUAL HEALING

In my first book, I included the Principles of Natural Healing—a list of eighteen principles I believe are the root of all we need to know and practice in holistic medicine. This list came to me in another vision I had after I signed my first book deal. The initial drafts weren't going so well—the text sounded too much like other books and theories that had been out there for eons. The deadline to submit the manuscript to the publisher was fast approaching, and I was getting increasingly desperate to find the breakthrough I needed to move forward.

Finally I said, "I need to get away so I can think!" I flew to Jamaica with my friend Darrel where we commenced three days of relaxing fun in the sun.

Fortunately, whatever was blocking my creative process was exorcised from my brain during those three days. On the morning of the fourth day in Jamaica, I told Darrel, "Leave me alone—go have a good time. Go running, go to the beach, hit the bars. I don't care. It's time for me to start my book."

I walked over to a cliff overlooking the ocean with a pad of paper, a pen, and a bottle of local Dragon Stout beer. I sat on a little white bench for maybe twenty or thirty minutes, hitting myself in the head in hopes of sparking a revelation. Everything I could think of to write was the same old, same old. My page was still blank, and I struggled to reach deep inside me for the answer.

As I watched the waves crash onto the rocks below, I asked myself, "What do you want to say that's so different? I know it's inside you."

After quite a few minutes more, and several more punches to the head and swigs out of my beer bottle, I picked up my pen, and like in the film *The Ten Commandments* by Cecil B. DeMille, the eighteen principles flowed out onto the pad of paper—one right after another. I didn't even think about what I was writing. It was as if I were being guided by some mysterious, unknown force. From that moment, with my principles to guide me, the book unfolded naturally—the roots of the entire book were contained in those eighteen principles.

As I worked to prepare the book you hold in your hands, another sixteen principles came to me, which I call the New Principles in the Spirit of Healing. These new principles aren't meant to replace the eighteen principles outlined in my first book—they are a supplement to them.

As you read through these principles, keep in mind that they apply just as much to our animal companions as they do to ourselves—especially in conjunction with the first eighteen principles in *The Nature of Animal Healing*.

1. My definition of science in the field of medicine is simply man trying to figure out what nature has already created.
2. With any degenerative condition, stability in the face of expected decline is actually improvement.
3. Hope consistently precedes healing.
4. Our companion animals are spiritual beings—perhaps more than we'll ever understand as humans.
5. When considering the big picture of existence and healing, spirituality is superior to physicality. This is more commonly expressed as "mind over matter."
6. The best solution is often the simplest one.
7. When designing programs to reestablish health, a vital ingredient in most all is *time*. Unlike the quick-fix goal of most conventional treatments, healing is a process that takes time.

   Corollary: Have patience with patients.
8. Before disease, there was health.
9. Disease is not something that just happens to you or

your animal companions, but something that you allow to happen, either consciously or unconsciously.

10. An illness is nature's way of creating the fundamental conditions necessary for healing called homeostasis.

11. Cancer is a confusion of nature caused mostly by man to now, in too many cases, outsmart himself.

12. The most predictable thing about cancer, patient to patient, is that it remains mostly unpredictable.

13. Health is not rocket science. Unfortunately, this is what medicine has become.

14. Our animal companions tell us what's wrong with them—we simply need to "listen" closely and openly.

15. The immune system functions at its best when it is in a completely unaltered state.

16. Everything necessary for healing is built into every living being. It's up to us to remove the obstacles to healing instead of adding new ones.

NEXT STOP BOULDER?

One of my best friends when I was in college at Cornell was Steve Rosdal. He graduated a year before I did and ended up working on Wall Street. After a couple years of that, he realized he couldn't carve out a good life doing what he was doing. So, he decided to escape from New York, move to Denver, and start over.

I always had a strong affinity for Colorado, especially Boulder. I thought it was an enlightened place to live and work, and its location right next to the Rocky Mountains was breathtaking. After I wrapped up my studies at Cornell and worked for a year in Horseheads, New York, I decided to move to Boulder and start a holistic veterinary clinic. I was serious. I began planning the move in earnest and I put in an order with the post office to have my mail forwarded to Steve's house in Denver. I was going to live with him while I scoped out the area.

Just days before my move date, however, my brother called and asked, "I want to give you my practice—would you like it?" My brother had the opportunity to buy a prestigious veterinary clinic in Bedford, which was more affluent and closer to where he lived. The veterinarian had died suddenly, and the practice went up for sale. The vet's widow was devastated, but she met my brother and sister-in-law, loved them, and offered to sell the practice to my brother. Once he took over the new practice, he would sell me his practice cheap.

I was excited by the offer—my brother had built an incredible reputation in the community as a veterinarian, and it would be a great opportunity for me because I would be able to run my own practice. At least that was the plan. My brother was supposed to put a down payment on the clinic on a Friday afternoon, but the widow was still distraught, and my brother didn't want to bug her about it over the weekend. Another veterinarian caught wind of the situation. He swooped in, gave the woman a down payment that weekend, and my brother lost out. I ended up joining my brother's practice, and I forgot all about making the move to Boulder. At that time I started to learn and practice the alternative treatments that became the foundation of my life's work.

BACK TO THE FUTURE

Much has changed in the twenty or so years since my first book was published. The kind of integrative veterinary medicine that I've been practicing during that time—and that almost cost me my license in the years before that book was published—has gained widespread acceptance. Alternative treatments for dogs and cats such as nutraceuticals and acupuncture are widely available if not yet commonplace, and society is beginning to understand that overvaccination is the root of many medical problems in our animal companions.

A company called Nutramax came out with the first well-known glucosamine supplement for humans, which is called Cosamin. Today, you can go to Costco and buy as much as you want of this "joint health" supplement. However, Nutramax eventually took a big step forward. They did a ton of research into treating animals with glucosamine and subsequently developed a supplement for dogs and cats called Cosequin, which is still widely available today. They put the science behind it, demonstrating that it works. Nutramax also created a supplement called Denamarin, and I estimate that at least half of all veterinarians prescribe it for animals with any kind of liver issue.

Slowly—as Cornell's CBD study clearly illustrates—the world of conventional veterinary medicine is waking up to the awesome potential of alternative treatments. These *are* the future of our field, and I'm extremely proud to have played a role in this transformation. It wasn't easy, and more than once I seriously considered retreating back to the comfort of the conventional medical establishment. But that just wasn't for me—I knew when I had my vision in Switzerland that my purpose was clearly laid out for me: to help save our favorite kingdom.

The ideas I wrote about in my first book were mostly my *opinions*—they didn't yet have a firm basis in science. But these opinions were so strong within me that I knew they were right, and I knew they needed to be shared. Today, they're no longer just my opinions—there is a large body of scientific and medical documentation on these treatments, on diet, on supplements, and on the inappropriateness of how we still standardly vaccinate. So, my role has changed from voicing my opinions into the void, to being a voice for the animals and a spokesperson for the available truth.

In this book, you'll learn the complete unvarnished truth as it exists today about the integrative veterinary practices that I pioneered, and that have opened the door for exploration by so many others into the vast field of alternative therapies. I will present the latest research—some of the university and pharmaceutical-company studies—and I'll take you to the leading edge of innovative, new treatments that you probably aren't yet familiar with. Throughout, I'll tell you a few of my own remarkable personal stories of animals and their people.

In the chapters that follow, I'm going to give you the latest advice, information, and treatment protocols that will help your animal companion live a longer and more fulfilling life. We'll cover everything from the basics of animal biology and psychology, to raw food, cancer, nutraceuticals, cutting-edge therapies, the spiritual connection we share with our dogs and cats—and much, much more.

Throughout, I look forward to opening your eyes to the tremendous power of nature, the spiritual world that our animal companions inhabit, and the role both these play within our human race.

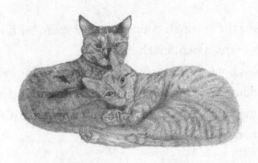

2

A NEW PERSPECTIVE ON HOW THE MIND AND BODY HEAL

The art of healing comes from nature, not the physician.
Therefore, the physician must start from nature,
with an open mind.
—Paracelsus

People have long wondered what it is within animals (particularly humans) that enables bodies to heal from most every kind of physical insult. We get cut, we bleed, we feel pain, but then—in just minutes—the bleeding stops. And within just a handful of days, our cut gets filled in with new tissue and we return to normal. Sure, we may have a scar to remember our date with the knife, but we're pretty much 100 percent again. Similarly, we can contract the flu and—after suffering days of fever and gastrointestinal turmoil—the majority of us bounce back from some extreme distress to good health.

Our animal companions are the same as us (no big surprise since we all sprang from the same source, many millennia ago). They get injured, they get ill. But, for the most part, they also heal—bouncing back from seemingly terrible circumstances. Physical trauma. Infections and sepsis. Cancer. Yes, cancer! I see it all the time in my practice.

What enables the mind and the body to heal? What is the remarkable power within us and our animal companions that shakes off serious injuries, illnesses, and diseases and returns us to normal? And what is the role of doctors, veterinarians, and other health practitioners in this process? Are they guides to healing or obstacles?

After graduating from the Cornell University College of Veterinary Medicine many years ago, I was a dyed-in-the-wool conventional veterinarian. When I examined ill or injured dogs or cats, my standard response was to prescribe conventional medications or surgical interventions—just as 99.9 percent of my colleagues routinely did. Unfortunately, many of the things we did to prevent or treat disease had side effects that caused more disease than what we were originally treating or trying to prevent. Although none of us wanted to inflict more damage on these animals, we felt we had no other choice. We had to live with collateral damage when using conventional therapies—it came with the turf.

As my veterinary experience grew, my eyes were opened to how the alternative therapies that worked so well for humans (some of which have been around for many thousands of years) could also be used successfully with dogs and cats. This led me to help pioneer integrative veterinary practice—merging the best of conventional and alternative medicine.

I understood that healing comes from nature—my job as a veterinarian was to support the tremendous healing power of nature, not get in its way.

But, unfortunately, getting in the way of nature's healing process is what common veterinary practice still dictates in so many cases. We overvaccinate our animal companions. We prescribe medications that cause side effects or that suppress natural healing. We do surgical and other procedures that should never be done. When I went to veterinary school, I was taught what I call the three Ds—how to how to Diagnose Disease and Drug it. Not until later did I learn how to channel the healing power of nature.

After I graduated from Cornell, I decided I wanted to stay in the area. A friend of mine—the president of my undergraduate fraternity—had taken a job at an animal hospital not far from where I lived. He was working with a well-established veterinarian. One day he called me and asked, "Hey, would you like to work with us? We can take it to a three-man practice."

The offer checked all the boxes. I would get to stay in my preferred location close to Cornell, and I would become an associate in a busy rural practice. I quickly agreed and was in business with my friend.

What I didn't realize at the time was that I was hired because my predecessor was dismissed after a parakeet in his care died under some unusual circumstances. A woman had brought her bird to the animal hospital to have his beak trimmed. The usual approach is to take a nail clipper and cut off the sharp point of the beak. It's usually a quick and easy procedure, but sometimes birds aren't too happy about it. This particular parakeet wasn't having it at all and thrashed around during the procedure.

Because of all the thrashing, when the veterinarian clipped off the point of the bird's beak, he cut off too much and it started to bleed.

To stop the bleeding, the veterinarian applied an electrocautery pen to the wound, which first required knocking out the bird with anesthesia. He took a plastic cone, packed it full of cotton, then poured on some ether—a highly volatile organic compound once commonly used as an anesthetic—and placed it over the parakeet's head. So far so good—the bird was out like a light.

That turned out to be a big mistake.

When the veterinarian touched the electrocautery pen to the parakeet's beak, it shot out an electrical spark and the bird exploded in the client's hand. Birds don't have lungs. Instead, they have air sacs through their bodies. The air sacs in this parakeet were filled with ether and became tiny bombs—detonating when the anesthesia was triggered by the spark. The veterinarian was fired immediately and that's how I got the job.

ASK DR. MARTY

Q: My dog is young and healthy and is eating a high-quality diet that is species appropriate. Does he still need to take supplements throughout his life?

A: This is a great question! In the not-too-distant past, animals got all the nutrition they needed through their natural diets. However, a variety of different things have gotten in between our animal companions and a natural diet. First, there has been an overall degradation of nutrition due to man's destruction of the natural content of the earth. The soil of our planet doesn't contain what it used to contain, and the fruits and vegetables that grow in that soil—and the humans and other animals that feed on these plants—don't contain the nutrients they used to contain. In addition, the pet food industry has adulterated much of our pets' diets—replacing much of the meat they should be eating with cereal and meat by-products (probably loaded with antibiotics and chemicals), with heat and intensive processing destroying much of whatever nutrients are left. Dogs and cats could live a long and healthy life just consuming the nutritiously rich food they naturally ate. This is sadly no longer the case. As the saying goes, "Let thy food be thy medicine"!

Nutritional deficiencies have taken their toll, compounded exponentially and genetically over many generations to where I consider hardly any domesticated companion animal to be born as healthy as nature intended. My true definition of a supplement then is a concentrated food to compensate for the deficiencies created in the food chain passed through the generations. A supplement, now called a nutraceutical, directly supplements the diet, which, in turn, indirectly supports the individual. You'll learn much more about supplements and nutraceuticals in chapter 5.

At the time, I lived in Ithaca in a tiny cottage and I commuted half an hour to the animal hospital. In 1973, there was a rock festival in Watkins Glen. It was scheduled for just one day and only three bands were booked to play—The Band, Grateful Dead, and Allman Brothers Band. While the plan was for a much-smaller event than Woodstock in 1969, the festival drew an estimated six hundred thousand people—far more than the four hundred thousand or so who attended Woodstock (including me!).

To get a good view of the stage, people jumped in their cars and trucks and vans and headed for the festival a couple days before the event was scheduled. As a result, the roads around Watkins Glen—a small town of just twenty-seven hundred people—were absolutely jammed. According to a report in *The Syracuse Post-Standard* at the time, Watkins Glen was "paralyzed by the onslaught of cars, trailers, campers, microbuses, trucks, and motorcycles." It reminded me of when I was at Woodstock and Arlo Guthrie announced to the crowd, "The New York State Thruway's closed, man!" The post office had to stop delivering mail, and the shelves of every store in the area were soon stripped bare.

On July 27—the night before the festival—I was at my cottage in Ithaca, on call for emergencies. Sure enough, I got an emergency call. Thirteen Saint Bernard puppies had maggots. I barely knew what a maggot was, but I definitely knew we had an emergency on our hands. So, I hopped in my car and turned south onto Route 13, a two-lane road that runs from Ithaca to Elmira, where the puppies were. Almost immediately, I was caught in a huge traffic jam. It usually took me just twenty-five minutes to get from Ithaca to Elmira, but

I was sitting at a near standstill for more than two hours. There were no cell phones—what was I going to do?

Eventually, I approached the fork in the road where you make a right to go to Watkins Glen or a left to go to Elmira. Everyone was headed to Watkins Glen, so I pulled onto the dirt shoulder to go around the cars that were trying to get to Watkins Glen. Keep in mind that, at the time, I looked like a freaking hippie with my long hair, beard, and army jacket. I didn't look much different from most of the young people on the highway that day going to the festival.

I was motoring along the dirt shoulder, trying to get to the Elmira turnoff, when a cop spotted my car and waved me over. "What the hell are you doing?" he demanded.

I looked at him. "I know you're not going to believe me, but I'm a veterinarian."

He cut me off. "And you have thirteen Saint Bernard puppies with maggots, right?"

An all-points bulletin had been put out on me. So he gave me a police escort to the hospital, and I was able to save all the puppies. When I first arrived, I wasn't sure exactly how I was going to treat the puppies—they were covered with maggots, even in their belly buttons and rectums. I picked some maggots off a puppy with tweezers and put them on the exam table. I exposed them to every antiseptic and disinfectant solution I could get my hands on. One of the solutions killed the maggots instantly. So, I took some sponges dipped in the solution and wiped down the puppies. The maggots quickly died, and I was left with thirteen very happy puppies—unharmed by the disinfectant.

A few months after my experience with the Saint Bernard puppies, my business partner Eddie signed up for an acupuncture course offered by a newly formed organization: the International Veterinary Acupuncture Society (IVAS). After taking the course, his mind was blown. To blow my mind, he put a dog on an exam table and asked me, "Do you want a stool sample?" He pushed a needle into an acupuncture point under the dog's rectum, intended to make the dog defecate. Suddenly, out of nowhere, a well-formed poop emerged.

As strange as it sounds, that changed my life right then and there. "Oh my God, I want to study acupuncture," I said. It was the most amazing thing I had ever seen. Eddie began integrating acupuncture into our practice. Hardly any veterinarians anywhere were offering acupuncture treatment, a new field, in the United States. I left the animal hospital after about nine months in preparation for my move to Denver to set up a holistic veterinary clinic in Boulder. That's when my brother offered me his practice in Westchester County, New York, and the rest is history.

One day, after having worked together for several months, we were having lunch when my brother asked me, "What do you *really* want to do?"

"I want to study acupuncture." I was excited by the prospect of merging together traditional and alternative veterinary practice. Becoming certified in veterinary acupuncture by the International Veterinary Acupuncture Society required participating in five four-day sessions over a series of long weekends that stretched over five months. Then you took the exam and hopefully passed and earned your certification. I had already missed the first two four-day sessions, so I called the IVAS office and asked, "Is there any way I can get in the certification course this year? I'll pay for the whole thing, take makeup sessions—whatever I need to do to get the training."

They said yes, but I would need to cram to make up the missed sessions, which I was happy to do. Earning my certification in veterinary acupuncture changed my life—more than anything else I had done in my practice.

The training took place in the Atlanta area and was accompanied by a Chinese acupuncture master, Dr. Ed Wong. In one demonstration, he showed us a basset hound that had been paralyzed for five months. When a dog is paralyzed for more than three weeks, the paralysis is considered to be permanent. And this dog was paralyzed—he was unable to use his back legs. But that wasn't all. The basset had been flown to Atlanta in the baggage hold of the aircraft. Unfortunately, the pressure in the baggage hold had dropped suddenly, and it was assumed that the basset hound's eardrums popped—leaving him both paralyzed *and* deaf. We could tell he was deaf because when Dr. Wong clapped his hands, the basset didn't respond.

Thirty or so students were in the class, and Dr. Wong had us all gather around the dog to get a close look at the acupuncture technique. He got to work, and the basset's hearing was instantly restored. We could tell because when Dr. Wong clapped his hands, the basset turned toward him. Dr. Wong placed some needles in the dog's back and legs, which he left there for about twenty minutes. The next morning, we went to class and the dog was walking—nowhere near normal, but he was definitely using his legs.

"What the hell is going on here?" I wondered.

The next session, we went to a farm somewhere outside Atlanta. The farmer brought out of the stall a horse that was chronically lame in one of his rear legs. Dr. Wong picked up the horse's hoof and pointed to a bulging vein. He asked for a 14-gauge needle. If you've never seen a 14-gauge needle, it's like a cannon. The higher the number, the smaller the bore of the needle. To give injections to animals, we use a 25- or 27-gauge needle. To take blood, we use a 20- or 21-gauge needle. The largest needles typically used in clinical practice are large-bore 16- and 18-gauge needles. Dr. Wong took the 14-gauge needle and stuck it in the horse's bulging blood vessel. Suddenly, a stream of blood shot out at least six feet from the end of the needle.

The blood formed a puddle. At first, the blood was a dark red. As he pointed to the stream of blood, Dr. Wong muttered, "Dark, dark." However, after about a liter of blood poured out of this horse's hoof, it turned bright red. Dr. Wong then muttered, "Red, red." He took the needle out of the horse's hoof and kept pressure on the spot for a couple of minutes so it wouldn't bleed. Then he let the horse run off, and it was no longer lame. It was completely normal. A month later, in our fifth and final session, we went out to the same farm to treat some of the other animals—dogs and cows. We asked the farmer how the horse was doing after the treatment, and he told us that the animal had been fine ever since. That added to the mind-blowing experiences in my education.

During the training, Dr. Wong took me aside. I was always the class clown, a real cutup, so I thought he was going to ask me to tone down my act. Instead, having an affinity for me, he asked, "What did they do in ancient China when a doctor's patient needed surgery?"

"Acupuncture," I spouted.

"No."

"Herbs, nutrition," I said a little less certainly.

"No."

"Then, what did they do?" I had no idea.

With great seriousness, Dr. Wong answered, "They killed the doctor because he was a failure to society."

Imagine the distance we have come from the natural-medical practice of ancient China, to modern-day technological medicine, where surgery, breast removal, cesareans, tumor removals, chemotherapy, and radiation are now routinely used to treat the diseases we have created. (Chemotherapy and radiation are two of the most powerful immunosuppressive agents known to medicine.) Why are we using things like these to treat diseases that are secondary to what these agents cause? We have strayed far from natural-medical practice. That's what I saw coming out of Cornell—the focus of conventional medicine is disease oriented: diagnose disease and drug it with powerful chemical agents that may actually cause disease.

We as doctors have learned relatively nothing about health care since ancient times. Our goal as physicians in modern medicine has been narrowly focused on disease treatment. That's where we went wrong as a profession.

How do you heal a cut? You clean it out and maybe put on a Band-Aid, right? But what if you don't—then what? Will you die? Do you have to sign onto Google? Absolutely not!

Nature has built powerful healing mechanisms into every animal, every living creature. It's already in there.

The immune system is at peak function when it's unadulterated, especially by man. Instead of focusing on diagnosing disease and drugging it, the focus should be on supporting the health and immune system of the patient. When you do that, you're providing the highest level of health care for the animals under your care. That's fundamental to the practice of integrative veterinary medicine, which I helped pioneer.

Why does nature create an inflammation? To sell cortisone? What's the purpose of a fever? Is it an aspirin deficiency? Of course not.

What I learned to do was to assign a purpose and a reason to disease, and to figure out why nature created it. What does the suffix -*itis* mean? It's inflammation. Nature creates inflammation to invoke the healing properties of the body. When you get punched in the eye or bang your elbow, it gets inflamed. We don't like that because inflammation creates symptoms or signs of disease and it hurts. It's uncomfortable. It takes you out of work. But we in the medical profession have learned how to drug that so you'll feel better faster. But, as I got deeper into my veterinary practice, I did a 180 and I started to assign purpose and reason for disease—working with disease to support it through its process instead of working against it.

When I lecture, I'll draw a swinging pendulum on the board to illustrate my transformation as a doctor. When I graduated from veterinary school, the pendulum was all the way up on the right side. I was ranked number two in my class early in my veterinary studies at Cornell, but I wasn't well physically. I was fighting a lot of health issues. Then I got into alternative medical practices—applying them to myself—and the pendulum swung all the way up the left side. I thought all conventional medicine was bad. I started to discount everything I learned in school.

When I realized that alternatives were the way to go for my own health, and that they also worked for animals in my veterinary practice, the pendulum started to swing less and less. Eventually it became balanced—right in between the two viewpoints of conventional and alternative practice. As amazing as acupuncture, herbs, and other alternative treatments were and are, I realized, "Hey, asshole, if you don't give this dog a shot of cortisone or antibiotics, it's going to die. If you don't remove this tumor, it's going to die." As much as I hate to use chemotherapy or surgery or radiation, I will choose it when it's needed to save the patient's life, and only then to buy us time to work on its immune system.

I've seen a huge misunderstanding during my career about what holistic medicine is. It is widely assumed that holistic medicine is the opposite pole to conventional medicine. However, true *holistic medicine*—a term I'm not fond of, I feel it's too airy-fairy—is the umbrella over both conventional and alternative medical practice, and it's what I have adopted over the years. A true holistic doctor will approach the body from both sides and provide what is needed holistically for that patient. This practice eventually became known as complementary medicine and then what it's called now: integrative medicine.

ASK DR. MARTY

Q: With all the controversy, what should a companion pet eat?

A: Realize that dogs and especially cats are carnivores and they evolved over eons to eat a predominantly fresh-meat diet. If your cat has ever proudly brought home a partially eaten mouse, you know this to be the case. Yes, things have changed through domestication, but looking especially at the teeth of dogs and cats and how pointy they still are—for eating meat, not grinding grain and cereals—you can easily see that this is still true. So, this is the direction you want to take in choosing the right diet for them. And it's important to know it is a *direction*, not an absolute. You're not just looking for that most ideal meal and then feeding your pet only that day in, day out, as the pet food industry would have you believe.

For humans, there are different levels of healthy eating, and most humans eat on many of those levels. We prefer to eat different combinations of meat, fish, vegetables, nuts, grains, dairy, and so forth with every meal. That provides us with a well-rounded diet that contains everything our bodies need to thrive. The same is true for pets. Know what's good for them (discussed in chapter 4) and "aim" in that direction. But, also, if they are basically healthy, variety is a key aspect of health and enjoyment of life for dogs and cats. Knowing these different levels, which ones to incorporate in their daily fare—and which ones to mostly avoid—should lead to a happy and healthy life for any pet.

In 2007, I attended a symposium, moderated by Dr. Mehmet Oz, for several hundred attendees at the Bravewell Collaborative in New York City. Before it shut down in 2015, the Bravewell Collaborative was at the forefront of advancing the practice of integrative medicine for humans. Dr. Oz was a celebrity by then—he had been a health expert on Oprah Winfrey's television show for a number of years, and a couple years later, Oprah produced *The Dr. Oz Show*, which became a hit. I had to take an early train to New York City for the event, and I arrived forty minutes before it was supposed to start. Coincidentally, as you'll read in chapter 10, I had successfully treated Oprah's dog Sophie some time earlier.

I wandered into the mostly empty ballroom, where tables were still being set up, and Dr. Oz was at the podium preparing. I had a bunch of my before-and-after case photographs with me because I had a meeting after this where I was going to show them. These photos showed ill dogs and cats before treatment, along with photos of the same animals healthy after treatment and pertinent medical records.

I had become a big fan of taking before-and-after photos even before I started my own veterinary practice. When I was still in school at Cornell, my girlfriend's roommate had a boyfriend, Kam, who was from Thailand. He taught me photography. I bought a Canon F-1 camera and became addicted to taking photographs. I became a good photographer with that camera.

As students, we used to go out to the local farms on ambulatory service to learn large-animal medicine—goats, horses, cows, pigs, and so forth. I would take my camera with me and take lots of photographs of the animals. I won the Cornell College of Veterinary Medicine Philanthropic Photography Award—$50 and a plaque. The $50 is long gone, but I still have the plaque on my wall. When I went into clinical practice, I took photos of everything of interest to me, which included before-and-after photos of all the animals I treated. They were often quite dramatic. Having those photographs, coupled with the often-hopeless cases that I turned around, had a tremendously positive impact on my career.

I started to get a buzz around the United States, and I would always show my before-and-after photographs in my presentations, coupled with the medical documentation. The more the word got out about my practice, the more people wanted me to treat their pets—the cases that other veterinarians had told them were hopeless. During an hour consult with these pet lovers, my goal was to start to educate them on why their animal was sick in the first place. I would show them the before-and-after photos. This would build up their hope. Not a false hope, but real hope that their dog or cat had a chance to recover and not die.

I went up to Dr. Oz—having no idea whether he would know who I was—and I said, "Hello, Dr. Oz. I know you've got a lot to do, but is there a chance I can talk with you after this is over? My name is Marty Goldstein."

Dr. Oz cut me off. "I know who you are. Oprah called me from her jet on the way to bring Sophie to see you. She asked me if she should keep on going or turn around. I was the one who told Oprah to continue on her way to see you."

Then he looked me in the eye, pointed his index finger

right at my nose, and said, "Do you know that Oprah loves you?"

I thought to myself, "You just won the lottery!"

Instead of meeting with me after the symposium, Dr. Oz told me he wanted to see what I had right then and there. We walked over to one of the tables, and I went through the before-and-after photos with him. He called the manager of his XM satellite-radio show and told him, "Book this man on my program!" One month later, I was a guest on his show for an entire hour.

Early one afternoon during the symposium I had lunch with Dr. Andrew Weil, and he told me about his own progression to an integrative view of medicine. He said, "Forget about calling it integrative medicine. It's just *one* medicine." Whatever you want to call it—holistic, integrative—it's the best of both worlds. The direction I want to take you and my profession in this book is that it's just *appropriate* medicine, or even better, *good* medicine.

Today, conventional medicine is opening up to the use of what were once alternative practices, including acupuncture and nutritional supplements. The pet food industry is going through a major upheaval, especially with the widespread availability of minimally processed raw and freeze-dried raw pet foods. Even the big guys are getting on board. Pet products giant Purina offers grain-free dog and cat food options and a bestselling probiotic. (We'll take a look later in this book at reports linking heart disease and grain-free pet foods.)

When treating difficult cases, I would usually have to work quickly and start the pets as soon as possible on supplements. But when a pet I saw came from the local area, I could take blood samples and start a more specific program in a couple days when the results were in. So, for example, if people came in on a Wednesday and we took blood samples from a person's pet, I'd ask the person to call me Friday morning to go through the results and get a program going ASAP. When people called, I'd first ask how their pet was doing. The response I received most often was "Oh, she's actually a bit better."

That's when it hit me. We hadn't even treated the patient yet, but we had changed the viewpoint of the animal's companion on disease. That's the spiritual connection—that's where we made a real difference.

I have a philosophy that pervades my veterinary practice. When you walk into a room that's pitch-black and you can't see where you're going, you don't try to destroy the dark. Just turn on a light. The same thing applies to an animal that is riddled with disease or cancer. You don't necessarily try to destroy that illness; you work on making the animal healthy. You turn on the light inside his body. You turn on a light inside his spirit. The spiritual relationship between human and animal is extremely powerful.

There's still so much we don't know about the working of the minds of both humans and our companion animals—and the depth of the bond between us. Researchers have found that dog and human genomes evolved together over thousands of years. In short, we share commonalities in our genetic structure as a result of our coevolution. According to the researchers, we share genes related to diet and behavior, diseases such as obesity, epilepsy, obsessive-compulsive disorder, and even some cancers. So, it's no accident that some of the so-called alternative treatments that work so well with humans are also quite effective with our animal companions. And vice versa.

I once treated a four-and-a-half-year-old cat named Fia, who was paralyzed due to an illness. Every single joint in her body, from the neck down, was fused together and immobile. Fia was sent to one of the largest specialty facilities in the Northeast, where she was diagnosed with a condition they called progressive fusing poly-osteoarthropathy. For two months, Fia was pumped full of steroids and two different kinds of antibiotics. There was no effect. In a last-ditch effort, they tried a two-week course of immune-suppressive chemotherapy. Still no effect. Finally, the veterinarians suggested to Fia's mom that they humanely end her animal companion's suffering.

That's when Fia was brought to me.

I assessed the case, and it was literally living rigor mortis. Every joint in Fia's body—except from her neck up—was rigidly fused. I wondered what had happened for Fia to reach this state and what I could do to help. My mind was a blank. I excused myself to go into my office. I sat down at my desk and gently hit my head with my hand, trying to come up with something, anything, that might help.

The only thing I could think of was to put her under deep, general anesthesia and try to mechanically break every frozen joint open with my hands. I had done this on pets with dislocated joints that had set improperly and were fusing that way. Then I would put Fia on injectable painkillers and have her mom sign a release form that if Fia woke up and I detected that she was seriously suffering, I could help her cross right then. But I didn't want to put her under general anesthesia immediately. I was concerned the drugs Fia was on were destroying her liver function, because that's what they do, and she wouldn't be able to wake up. So, I asked Fia's mom to give me another seven to ten days.

I took a blood sample so I could work on a program, and I gave Fia an injection of a homeopathic remedy from Germany called Zeel. No steroids, no antibiotics, and no immune-suppressive chemotherapy. Then I sent Fia home with a remedy and a supplement for joint problems. By the time her mom was driving from New York back to New Jersey, Fia was walking around in the car.

How did the treatment make Fia walk? I don't know. If you look at what a homeopathic remedy is, it's less than one part per billion or trillion. If you brought that remedy to a sophisticated scientific laboratory, nothing would be found on analysis but sterile saline. Homeopathy is an amazing science that is so little understood by conventional medicine. There's not much difference between the vibrational aspect of a homeopathic remedy and the frequency of spiritual thoughts. Imagine what power a positive thought could have on healing.

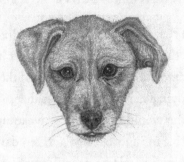

3

INSIDE YOUR PET'S MIND AND BODY

I am fond of pigs.
Dogs look up to us. Cats look down on us.
Pigs treat us as equals.
—WINSTON CHURCHILL

Deciding on the best approaches for maintaining the good health of our animal companions requires a basic knowledge of the workings of their minds and bodies. While mammals share many characteristics (scientists say that we humans share about 84 percent of our genome with dogs,[1] 90 percent with cats—and 60 percent with bananas),[2] dogs and cats are different from us humans in many significant ways. Before we get into the specifics, let's take a trip back in time—a *very* long trip back.

If you turn back the clock far enough, you'll find that humans, dogs, and cats share a common ancestor. While there's been quite a lot of research and debate on the topic over the years, it's thought by scientists that the first "true" mammal (placental like humans, versus marsupial like kangaroos or egg laying like platypuses) emerged around 160 million years ago. This now-extinct animal, given the scientific name *Juramaia sinensis,* was a small (about half an inch long, and weighing perhaps half an ounce or so), furry creature that ate insects and worms and looked a bit like a shrew.[3] Aside from being placental, what set it apart from other mammals at the time was its ability to climb trees, which gave it a tremendous competitive advantage—both in locating food sources and in self-protection.

Fast-forward many millions of years to a time when dogs and cats had developed as creatures quite different from their distant, shrewlike ancestors. Research shows that today's dog evolved from wolves, while what we know today as cats evolved from wild cats. It's thought that dogs became domesticated approximately fifteen thousand years ago, while cats became domesticated about ten thousand years ago. Since that time, we have been fast friends and companions.

We as humans share much with our dog and cat companions besides our homes, our beds, our living room sofas, and our cars. Aside from the obvious biological similarities (warm-blooded metabolisms, which allow us to maintain our body temperature relatively constant in spite of our environment, four-chambered hearts, hair, mammary glands, and so on), dogs and cats are intelligent, have unique personalities, are social, express a variety of different emotions, can learn, and can communicate—verbally and nonverbally, with each other, and with us humans. As every dog and cat lover knows, we can form remarkably deep and strong bonds of friendship, loyalty, and even love—often for a lifetime.

I became attuned to the similarities between dogs and cats and humans many years ago when I started a crusade to improve my health. What I tried on me, I tried on dogs and cats. What worked for me, worked for them, too. When I began my schooling in acupuncture for animals with the International Veterinary Acupuncture Society, a veterinarian, Dr. Norman Ralston, was invited to give a lecture to our class. Norman was a pioneer. He started doing holistic and integrative veterinary medicine—and I think acupuncture—back in the 1950s.

The topic of his lecture was improving the health of dogs using a macrobiotic diet. I was also eating a macrobiotic diet, which I had found improved my health. Dr. Ralston told us that the proper recipe for the macrobiotic diet for dogs was quite simple: 50 percent brown rice, 25 percent beef, and 25 percent green, leafy vegetables. This simple diet worked wonders because the quality of the food was so much better than what the vast majority of dogs were getting. The most popular pet foods then were highly processed, full of chemicals, and low in nutrition.

Before we started learning about the importance of diet for animal health, we fed our dogs Gaines-burgers and Top Choice. Consider the chemistry set of twenty-eight ingredients that used to be found in each and every Gaines-burger and compare it to the three wholesome food ingredients in Dr. Ralston's recommended macrobiotic diet for dogs:

- Soybean meal
- High fructose corn syrup
- Soybean grits
- Cornmeal germ
- Meat
- Water sufficient for processing
- Corn syrup
- Propylene glycol
- Animal fat preserved with BHA
- Calcium carbonate
- Phosphoric acid
- Vegetable oil preserved with BHA and citric acid
- Salt
- Potassium sorbate (a preservative)
- Sodium carboxymethylcellulose
- Artificial color
- Ferrous sulfate
- Zinc oxide
- Vitamin E supplement
- Vitamin A supplement
- Vitamin B12 supplement
- Copper oxide
- Calcium pantothenate
- Vitamin D supplement
- Ethylenediamine dihydriodide
- Riboflavin supplement
- Thiamin mononitrate
- Pyridoxine hydrochloride

Is it any wonder that Gaines-burgers had the mysterious power to stay moist and red in a dog's bowl for the better part of an entire week? How could this "food" be considered real—or healthy?

I began feeding my dogs a wholesome home-cooked macrobiotic diet—the same one I myself had adopted—and added a small selection of supplements, including vitamins A and D, vitamin E, B complex, and vitamin C. Eventually, I started adding sesame and safflower oil, and maybe some cod-liver oil, which was my source of vitamin A. Dosing was based on what I would personally take. So, a 150-pound human would take a certain dose of vitamin C, and a 50-pound dog got one-third of that. The dogs responded well to this supplemented diet—far beyond expectations.

This was my epiphany, and the start of my own journey—transforming what I learned from the human mammal kingdom and applying it to the broader animal mammal kingdom. The animals became noticeably healthier from this diet; sometimes the difference was night and day. Their eyes glowed. Theirs coats were thicker and shinier, and no longer had that dull, waxy look and feel. Their mood and mobility were much improved, and even their breath changed for the better.

As I started to go to health food stores, I learned more about the multitude of supplements available besides those basic vitamins that I was using. When a supplement sounded incredible—say some vitamin, mineral, or herb—I would use it on dogs and even cats, giving them an appropriate dose according to their weight. The more I worked on my own health, the more I also started to apply common sense to the animals.

When I lecture to veterinarians, I always say, "I have two associates that are by far the most effective of all the doctors that I consult with, and those two associates are called *nature* and *common sense*. You have those, too. Don't feel you have to do everything by what you learned in the four years of medical school—use common sense, and respect what nature is doing in the body."

I teach this same philosophy to my clients. People are so dependent on getting a doctor's opinion when they should also be listening to and trusting their own wisdom. I tell them, "This is *your* companion—someone that you've lived with for years. You know his or her moods and habits. When a veterinarian sees your dog or cat, it might be for just a half hour at a time. Don't be afraid to use your own judgment, and especially feeling." I believe that this is the best path for everyone who is blessed to have an animal companion in life.

When I first started my practice, there was just one supplement for pets—Pet-Tabs, a multivitamin and mineral supplement put out by Beecham Massengill that is still produced by Zoetis. There were also all those unhealthy chemicals and synthetic additives in good old Gaines-burgers, Top Choice, Alpo, Ken-L Ration, and the rest of the products sold by the large pet food companies. Today, a zillion supplements are available for animals, which creates mass confusion for consumers. I'm probably aware of just 15 to 20 percent of the supplements available right now, even though I've been giving animals supplements for longer than almost anyone else in the United States. Why? Because there are so many of them.

Although you can do as I did way back, all sorts of supplements are now specifically formulated for pets, and they have proper dosing by weight on their labels. The best thing you can do is to always consult with a veterinarian well experienced in integrative medical practice. You can find a qualified veterinarian near you—and the modalities they practice—by visiting the American Holistic Veterinary Medical Association website: https://www.ahvma.org.

The next step in my journey—after adapting my own macrobiotic diet with vitamin supplements for dogs and cats—was to start using symptom-oriented supplements, such as glucosamine sulfate to treat joint and related structural problems. Then, in 1978, a client told me a group of veterinarians were saying that my license should be suspended because I was treating arthritic dogs with glucosamine sulfate and was not using standard medical therapy. Ironically, approximately $636 million in pet supplements are now sold each year—a significant portion of which is composed of glucosamine sulfate.[4] Research shows that one-third of all US households with dogs use supplements, along with one-fifth of all US households with cats. According to a report by market-research firm Packaged Facts:

> Joint health supplements remain the most commonly purchased condition-specific pet supplement according to Packaged Facts' January 2015 survey of pet owners, followed by those supporting heart health and skin and coat health, then digestive health/hair-

ball prevention, and omega fatty acid supplements. Probiotics, senior formula supplements, and omega fatty acid supplements were more popular with cat owners, while more dog owners than cat owners give their pets joint health supplements.[5]

I decided to use symptom-oriented supplements because of the similarities in the different mammalian species— humans and dogs and cats. But there are distinct differences, too. First, dogs and cats are carnivores—we humans are not. Even though dogs, through domestication, have strayed from strict carnivority and are now considered omnivores, cats are obligate carnivores—*true* carnivores. If you look at any dog's mouth and tooth structure, there is not one tooth flat for grinding cereal or grain (which is why humans' molars are flat). Also, and very important, is that the stomach of a dog is thicker and more muscular for the initial digestion and processing of meat and bones. The hydrochloric acid concentration is stronger in a dog's stomach than a human's, to digest the protein of meat and bones rather than the alkaline diet that humans are normally supposed to have.

In addition, the intestinal tract of dogs is shorter than ours compared to body weight. Let's say you take some vegetables and brown rice and put them in a pail at 100°–102°—roughly the same as the internal body temperature of a dog measured rectally. They will start to rot. Now, take some meat and allow it to rot at the same temperature. Which do you think is going to stink worse after a few days? The meat, because it goes so foul. A dog's intestinal tract is shorter than ours so the meat will pass through with minimal putrefaction. That's why humans on high-meat diets have so many problems. The meat gets stuck in there because the intestine is a lot longer, and it putrefies.[6]

Now the other big thing—which is the foundation of my work over the years—is that when dogs and cats kill their prey, they eat the organs and not just the muscle. Most processed pet foods (remember the list of ingredients for those Gaines-burgers?) ignored this (and still do)—making the diets of our animal companions organ deficient. So, my next step after getting the animals on a macrobiotic diet, and adding in vitamin A, vitamin C, vitamin D, vitamin B, and then symptom-oriented supplements such as glucosamine sulfate and high levels of oil (especially when they had skin problems), was glandular supplements. This was based on the work of an absolute genius, Dr. Royal Lee. In the 1940s, he laid down the entire theory and thesis of how to analyze blood metabolically, leading to the prescription of certain nutraceuticals, but especially concentrated glandular supplements.

When we started to add glandular supplements for animals, our success rate skyrocketed—they responded so incredibly well. More resistant cases we worked on suddenly responded positively with this simple addition to their diet. Even though Dr. Lee laid down glandular supplements for humans, it just made more sense to do it with animals because that's what they ate in nature.

Long story short, these and other differences inform what humans, dogs, and cats should eat to maintain optimum health. We'll dive much deeper into this topic in the next chapter.

ASK DR. MARTY

Q: Why is there so much cancer now in our companion animals?

A: The incidence of cancer in our pets, and how much it has escalated during the span of my career as a practicing veterinarian, is alarming. Although much mystery and complexity surround this multitrillion-dollar-a-year industry called cancer, the foundation is simple. Cancer occurs when the immune system no longer controls the proper differentiation of cells from their stem cell roots into normal, functioning cells. So, if we want to therapeutically stop cancer cells from growing or prevent that in the first place, our focus needs to be on immune system health—stopping what suppresses or impedes its proper function—and not just on "cancer."

A FLOOD OF PERCEPTION

We're all familiar with the standard categories of senses that most members of the human race share: sight, hearing, smell, taste, and touch. Through these five senses (and perhaps some others that we'll explore later in this section) our brains make sense of the world around us.

The absence of any of these five senses can cause all sorts of challenges for us. The absence of sight makes a simple walk through the woods difficult, though certainly not impossible. If we can't hear, we need sign language (perhaps in combination with lipreading) to communicate effectively with others. If our sense of smell is defective, we can't tell if the food we are about to eat is rotten or contaminated, and we can become ill as a result. If we have lost our sense of taste, we can't enjoy to the fullest tomorrow evening's visit to our favorite restaurant. Without the sense of touch, we wouldn't feel pain when picking up a hot pan or stepping into a scalding-hot shower, and we could be seriously injured.

We share all five of these senses with dogs and cats (and many other animals). But what if I told you that there are actually more than fifty perceptions, and that we also share these with our friends in the animal kingdom? While some of these are things you would never think of as perceptions, and you might not be consciously aware of them, I believe they exist, and most play a significant role in our lives.

We have the inherent ability, for example, to perceive color, the relative sizes of objects, and pitch, tone, volume, and rhythm. We can certainly perceive the emotions of others, both individuals and groups, and we can detect hormonal signals—pheromones—that other humans release into the environment in a variety of different endocrine states. We can sense the physical energy of others, the position and movement of our body and joints (proprioception), compass direction, and more.

The perception of time plays a major role in our lives and in the lives of our animal companions. We humans may live sixty, eighty, even a hundred years. Dogs and cats may live ten or fifteen years. As a result, time is exaggerated in their universe. So, if you get a dog that is terminal with cancer to live three more years, it's like getting a human maybe up to a couple more decades of life.

Most of us have heard (and probably believe) that one year in the life of a dog is equal to seven years in the life of a human. That's not exactly true, because the progression of time for a dog is not the same as it is for a human. As pointed out in a *New York Times* article from some years ago, the first year of a dog's life is equivalent to roughly fifteen years in the life of a human—not seven.[7] In addition, the size of a dog has a bearing on age for dogs, with large dogs aging faster than smaller dogs. Here are some figures that WebMD put together to show just how old dogs are in human years as they age:[8]

THE AGE OF YOUR DOG IN HUMAN YEARS			
DOG SIZE	SMALL	MEDIUM	LARGE
AGE OF DOG	AGE IN HUMAN YEARS	AGE IN HUMAN YEARS	AGE IN HUMAN YEARS
1	15	15	15
2	24	24	24
3	28	28	28
4	32	32	32
5	36	36	36
6	40	42	45
7	44	47	50
8	48	51	55
9	52	56	61
10	56	60	66
11	60	65	72
12	64	69	77
13	68	74	82
14	72	78	88
15	76	83	93
16	80	87	120

The way dogs and cats perceive barriers and the solids in our physical universe is interesting, too. We humans get far more upset if some obstacle gets in our way than they do. They'll go around it, they'll jump over it, or they'll back off if necessary. They just deal with it, whereas humans tend to internalize it.

While humans don't seem to be particularly attuned to magnetic fields, many other animals definitely are. Later in this book, we'll explore pulsed electromagnetic field (PEMF) therapy, which I am convinced is the medicine of the future. NASA has conducted extensive studies on this therapy,[9] and Dr. Oz has been exploring it as well. But what's really interesting, especially with horses, is if you turn the machine on, the animal will go over to it and put its hurt leg against the device. Animals have a greater perception of magnetic fields than we do—perhaps because there's so much noise, distraction, and interruption in our human environment that we tend to tune it out.

It should be no great surprise that animals in general (including, to a lesser extent, humans) are attuned to such things as magnetic fields. I'm fascinated by something called the Schumann resonance. In short, because of electrical activity in the earth's atmosphere, electromagnetic waves are created that bathe the planet and every living thing that resides on it. We're conceived in these waves, we're born in these waves, we live in these waves, and we die in them. The fundamental Schumann resonance occurs at a frequency of 7.83 Hz (or cycles per second), while progressively weaker resonances also occur at 14.3, 20.8, 27.3, and 33.8 Hz.

The fundamental Schumann resonance at 7.83 Hz is the resonant frequency of the earth's atmosphere, and many observers consider this to be the frequency of life itself. Though it's not something we are consciously aware of (the best ears in the world can only hear sounds that have a frequency of 20 Hz or higher), it affects our health and well-being—it might be at their very root.

Experiments conducted by Dr. Luc Antoine Montagnier—who discovered the human immunodeficiency virus and was awarded the Nobel Prize in physiology for his work—found that DNA sequences communicate with each other via low-frequency electromagnetic waves. The frequency on which these DNA sequences communicate? 7.83 Hz. We'll take a closer look at this and the related science in chapter 6.

The point of this discussion is that there is much more to healing and our relationship with the animal kingdom than meets the eye, ear, nose, tongue, and skin—the nodes of the traditional five senses.

AN INTENSE LEVEL OF SPIRITUAL COMMITMENT

I'm always amazed, but never surprised, by the intense level of spiritual commitment people have for their animal companions. The relationship goes much deeper than just companionship or affection. Years ago, a couple—Larry Canova and his wife, Lana—hired a jet to fly their German shepherd named King to me from California, north of Los Angeles.

It cost them $16,000 to fly the dog across the country. King had a tumor on the top of his skull. I called in my favorite surgeon—Dr. Martin DeAngelis—to assist. He's one of the most accomplished surgeons in the history of veterinary medicine, and he served as chief of orthopedics and acting head of surgery at the Animal Medical Center in Manhattan, which is the largest nonprofit animal hospital in the United States, with more than a hundred veterinarians in seventeen specialties all under one roof—and an imposing eight stories tall.

Ironically, when my license was being threatened and I was trying to stay out of the limelight, Martin represented to me the epitome of conventional veterinary practice because of his position at the Animal Medical Center. Then, one day, my brother and I were at our clinic in Yorktown Heights when I looked over the front desk into the waiting room and there he was, sitting in a chair. I ran back to the room where my brother was, looking as if I had seen a ghost.

My brother looked at me. "What's wrong?"

"We're screwed."

"What do you mean?"

"Martin DeAngelis is sitting in the waiting room!" I was convinced he had brought with him a claim from the American Veterinary Medical Association (AVMA).

"Just be cool," my brother told me. "Talk with him and don't make a scene."

I invited Dr. DeAngelis into an examination room, and he brought along a cat carrier. Inside the carrier was a seventeen-year-old cat named Jersey. Dr. DeAngelis had previously surgically removed a fibrous tumor from the side of Jersey's abdomen, but the tumor had grown back. He asked, "Should I cut her again? I'm here because I want your opinion."

I was trying to be as cool as I could be—doing whatever I could to maintain a medical-professional demeanor—but I was still recovering from the shock of having this veterinary icon in our clinic. I told him, "I wouldn't recommend doing another surgery—you can't do better than you did the first time, and she's also seventeen years old. Instead, I would put her onto nutritional supplements."

Dr. DeAngelis followed my recommendation, and Jersey's tumor shrank. This outcome changed DeAngelis's life. His wife, Kathi, one the most gifted artists I personally know, also turned to the healing arts. Martin discovered an entirely new world of therapies and treatments that aren't conventional or approved by the AVMA. I've brought him in to do surgery ever since—he has the uncanny ability to perform remarkable surgeries on animal companions whose cases are far beyond hopeless. He also now realizes that surgery doesn't cure disease—it just addresses a symptom. It's one part of an integrative care regimen that encompasses a variety of different modalities.

The surgeon's motto is "A chance to cut is a chance to cure," and we know that's not entirely true. For example, while some tumors are encapsulated with firm boundaries and can completely and relatively easily be removed, others are widely spread with no defined boundaries. This makes it remarkably difficult for a surgeon to completely remove the tumor and ensure it won't just grow back. Even with well-encapsulated tumors, removal doesn't get to the root of the problem—what caused the tumor. It's also extremely frustrating to the surgeon who wants to do everything he or she can to cure the patient once and for all.

This was certainly the case with Martin, who always wanted the best outcomes for his patients but couldn't always get the entire tumor out. In those cases, I would tell him, "Just do your best—remove as much as possible. I'll work on the immune system." It wasn't uncommon for us to do a follow-up exam a few months later and find that the tumor was totally gone.

So, back to my story about King, the German shepherd. I called Martin in to do surgery with me. We opened up the dog's skull, and Martin removed as much of the tumor as he possibly could. I then performed cryosurgery to help attain a more favorable long-term outcome by destroying more of the cancer we could not get to by conventional means. We put King's skull back together, and after a short recovery period, the Canovas flew him back home on the private jet—bringing the round-trip transportation costs alone up to $32,000.

Sadly, the tumor grew back, and the Canovas decided to have us do a follow-up surgery—flying him out again on the private jet. We opened King's skull and I looked at the top of his brain. Martin cut out the new growth, I again performed cryosurgery, and we buttoned everything up. When it was time to fly King back home, the Canovas boarded the jet with him—and they waited and waited, as the weather delayed their getting out of Westchester County Airport. They sat on the tarmac for more than two hours, until finally they got the okay to take off.

As they started taxiing down the runway, Lana yelled out, "There's something wrong with King!"

King's abdomen was severely bloated, a sure sign that he had gastric torsion, which is when a dog's stomach twists and overstretches due to excess gas pressure. It's thought this acute condition has a genetic component, and dogs with deep chests—including German shepherds and Great Danes—are particularly susceptible to it. Even if you catch it in time and it's surgically corrected, the damage may be so extensive that the patient dies anyway.

Larry jumped out of his seat, ran up to the pilot, and shouted, "Stop the plane!"

The plane stopped halfway down the runway and was brought back to the terminal, and the Canovas got on the phone with Dr. DeAngelis, who lived in New Paltz—about an hour and a half away. They all met up at the Westchester Rockland emergency clinic that I used to work at after I sold my last practice. DeAngelis did the surgery—opening up King's abdomen and untwisting his stomach. The plane flew back to Los Angeles with no one on it—racking up another $16,000. Eventually, the Canovas did get King back home.

But the story isn't over yet—the tumor grew back again. I knew we had to find a real solution, not just remove it over and over, especially since Larry would not give up trying.

So, I called my dear friend Dr. George Zabrecky, who is the most brilliant man I know in human integrative medicine. He told me about a therapeutic agent developed in Russia called Radachlorin, used in photodynamic therapy. It's a photosensitizer made of chlorophyll extracted from *Spirulina* algae, and it has been used to fight a variety of different cancers. When you inject Radachlorin intravenously, it gets sucked up by the tumor because of its high ammonia content. You then shine a special light—which emits a specific wavelength of light tuned to the color of the Radachlorin—on the tumor site. The Radachlorin in the tumor absorbs the light, which causes it to degrade rapidly because of the flood of free radicals released as a result of the therapy.

So, based on George's recommendation, Larry Canova bought several vials of Radachlorin and one of the special General Electric lights for $5,400. We injected the Radachlorin, and two hours later we put King under anesthesia. We then positioned the light over King's skull, keeping it in place for forty-five minutes. The tumor became bright red and inflamed, and the next day it was smaller.

Long story short, King did sadly finally succumb to his illness. We did everything we could possibly do to help him—and the Canovas spent a total of $96,000 ($134,000 in today's dollars) in travel expenses alone, flying him from one side of the country to the other for treatment—but some illnesses just can't be cured. It's in God's hands, or in the hands of some higher power. As doctors, we must acknowledge and accept that.

One day Lana was cleaning out the house and found the light we used to treat King. She told her husband, Larry, that she was going to take the light to the local FedEx. As she walked out the door, Larry demanded, "Where are you going to send that light?!"

"I'm sending it to Dr. Marty so he can continue to use it in his research."

"That's the light that killed King!"

Lana turned around and looked her husband in the eye. "Larry, I thought it was cancer that killed King."

And Lana was right.

THE GMOS AND GLYPHOSATE

Jeffrey Smith is a consumer advocate who is particularly concerned about the presence of genetically modified organisms (GMOs) and glyphosate in our food, and in the food of our animal companions. In 2019, I had the good fortune to meet Jeffrey in person at the Truth About Cancer conference in Anaheim, California, where we were both invited to speak. Read his following sidebar to learn more about why we should be concerned about what the dogs and cats in our lives are eating.

ARE WE POISONING OUR PETS WITH GMOS AND GLYPHOSATE IN PET FOODS?

BY JEFFREY M. SMITH

Executive Director, Institute for Responsible Technology

In the late 1990s, the nationally syndicated "Animal Doctor" columnist, Dr. Michael Fox, received alarming letters from pet owners around the country. Out of the blue, their dogs and cats were struck with diarrhea, itchy skin, and other persistent disorders. Dr. Fox had a theory.

Genetically modified organisms (GMOs) had just been introduced into both the human and pet food supply. Specifically, genes from bacteria had been inserted into the genomes of several food crops such as soy and corn. Many experts, including scientists working at the US Food and Drug Administration (FDA), had tried in vain to warn of possible health effects and stop the introduction.

Dr. Fox wrote back to the pet owners, asking that they immediately switch to pet foods that did *not* use GMOs. He later filled a file cabinet with their thank-you notes. His recommendation worked beautifully.

I've spoken with many veterinarians who have also connected the dots of animal disease to GMOs in food. Some change the animals' diets before doing anything else and report that most of the issues are resolved or managed without further treatment.

We began tracking similar changes in humans a decade ago. I had presented the research on GMO health dangers at numerous medical conferences, and as a result thousands of physicians began prescribing non-GMO and organic diets to their patients. What I later heard from these doctors blew my mind. A significant percentage of their patients had dramatic recoveries. The docs were 100 percent convinced that GMOs were a major driver of disease.

I started asking audiences at my lectures, "What health improvements, if any, did you notice after switch-

ing to non-GMO and organic diets?" With each tes-
timonial, I asked the room, "How many others noticed
improvement in this condition?" In 150 talks, I heard the
same results over and over.

Eventually, our nonprofit Institute for Responsible
Technology (IRT) surveyed subscribers and received responses from 3,256 people. They reported pretty much
the same thing I heard in the lectures: improvement in
twenty-eight conditions, many disappearing entirely.

An additional eighty respondents, however, filled out
the questionnaire on behalf of their pets. As the chart
below shows, the conditions that improved in pets also
improved in humans. Both had digestive health as the top
benefit.

% of respondents reporting improved health conditions after humans and pets switched to a non-GMO and mostly organic diet

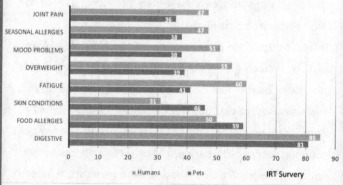

There are many reasons why GMOs may be responsible for these and other disorders. For example, most

GMOs are engineered to survive otherwise deadly sprays of Roundup weed killer. This makes weeding easier for farmers but may be killing humans and animals.

Glyphosate is the primary toxin in Roundup. In 2015, it was officially named a probable human carcinogen by the World Health Organization's International Agency for Research on Cancer. There weren't enough studies on people to call it definite. But there *were* sufficient studies to confirm that it definitively causes cancer in animals.[10]

IRT recently tested popular pet foods for glyphosate levels. The results were shockingly high. This helps explain the finding by the Health Research Institute (HRI) that dog urine averages an astounding forty times more glyphosate than human urine. Cats also have higher glyphosate levels than humans, though not as high as dogs'.

Soon after glyphosate began being used on our food, cancer in dogs and cats began to skyrocket. We don't think this is a coincidence.

Roundup is not only sprayed on the Roundup Ready GMOs, including soy, corn, cotton, canola, sugar beets (not table beets—just those used for sugar), and alfalfa. It is also used to dry down (desiccate) other varieties of crops just days before harvest. Grains are often sprayed, including oats, wheat, barley, and others. Legumes such as lentils and beans are also sprayed. And glyphosate is used near numerous fruits and vegetables. The highest levels of glyphosate residues are found in chickpeas, lentils, pea products, soy, and oats.

Both GMOs and the Roundup sprayed on these crops

are not just linked to cancer. They have been implicated in a long list of disorders. GMO animal studies reveal organ damage, premature death, tumor formation, immune system damage, birth defects, infertility, and other serious issues. The research on Roundup and glyphosate is more extensive. The toxin appears to damage the balance of the essential microorganisms in our digestive tract (microbiome), inhibit the production of key compounds needed for brain chemistry and liver detoxification, throw off the delicate balance of hormones, inhibit the cell's production of energy, create leaky guts with gaps between the cell walls, promote birth defects, and cause cancer.

The good news is that organic products are not allowed to intentionally contain GMOs or Roundup. Purchasing organic food for you and your pet is a great way to minimize exposure. A few nonorganic brands also avoid GMOs and glyphosate use.

Also, make sure those maintaining the lawns and parks where your animals roam are alerted to this threat, so they don't use Roundup to kill weeds. It can easily be absorbed through paws and transferred from the hair of pets who roll on the ground to kids and adults who pet them.

Go to www.PETSandGMOS.com for a list of tested pet foods with glyphosate levels and recommendations of pet foods that don't allow GMOs and glyphosate in their production. At www.ResponsibleTechnology.org, you can get a list of glyphosate levels in human food. And at www.RoundupRisks.com, learn how to approach the decision makers who can stop the use of Roundup on parks and public lands.

ALKALINE WATER—YES OR NO?

Although there are many similarities between us and our companion dogs and cats, I feel one major difference is worth considering. I know with humans that we should be eating a diet that's basically alkaline in nature, or, more specifically, one that keeps the body alkaline. One of the healthiest things I do to restore my health is an alkalizing citrus purge that I learned from one of the all-time favorite health experts, N. W. Walker.

Also, in-home alkaline water systems have gained much popularity. I have had many people over the years inquire about giving their pets alkaline water. I am not opposed to this and have heard people claim their pets do well on it. But here's my conundrum. One of the number one things that people eat, besides sugar and processed carbs, that acidify the body is meat. Our pets are carnivores and should be eating mostly a meat diet, which is acidifying.

In blood sample results, one of the most important is the level of an enzyme called alkaline phosphatase. It is made in the liver but metabolically references the functioning of the adrenal glands, which take care of stress and inflammation. This enzyme also commonly elevates with chronic degenerative disease, especially of joints and bones and with cancer. Look at the name of this enzyme, *alkaline phosphatase*. When its levels elevate in the blood, then the blood is too "alkaline."

So, do we want to give pets something *more* alkaline? I don't know the answer to this, and more research is needed.

In the meantime, however, a more natural way of balancing the alkalinity and acidity of your animal companion's diet is through the addition of a small amount of fresh fruits and vegetables. This is the way nature intended your dog to eat a balanced diet—not by buying an alkaline water system.

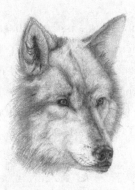

4

FOOD IS STILL WHERE IT STARTS

Do not put chewed bones back on plates. Instead,
throw them on the floor for the dog.
—DESIDERIUS ERASMUS

In my first book, I wrote about the critically important role of diet to our animal companions' good health. Most pet parents had been sold on the idea that simply opening a can of Ken-L Ration or a bag of Purina Dog Chow or Friskies and putting the contents into a dog's or cat's food bowl was sufficient—that everything necessary for their pet's good health would be found within that can or bag. Today we know that this is definitely not the case.

The pet food industry has undergone a remarkable transformation over the past decade, as has our knowledge of what constitutes a truly good diet for our animal companions, and what does not. There have been tremendous advances in the pet food industry, but the most important is that we have taken a big step backward to what our pets really should be eating. Before we explore the food that dogs and cats need for optimum health and a happy and long life, let's take a look at how pet food has evolved over time, and how we got to where we are today.

When I wrote my first book back in 1999, I fed my companion animals mostly food that I personally cooked for them. It was simple, wholesome, and healthy. When it comes to what food is best to feed dogs and cats, however, there has been a significant change of opinion. I predicted this change more than twenty years ago in this line taken from page 61 of my first book:

> On the issue of raw food for pets, I've recently gone from wary endorsement to real enthusiasm. . . . And seeing the effects that an increase in raw food has on animals has led me to increase the amount of it for my pets as well as in my own diet. I fully expect all the members of my household to be living *exclusively* on raw foods.[1]

Yes, the health and well-being and happiness of our companion animals really does all begin with food. I believe that a major aspect of how chronically or generally ill our companions have gotten over my career began with the degradation of the food chain. It worsened as we humans changed our opinions on how best to feed a dog or a cat. As I've always said, if the pet food industry had originally been created by scientists who actually studied the ways dogs and cats eat in nature, we would never have created the nutritional wasteland that commercial pet food became.

Let's take a quick look at how we got to our current place.

THE EMERGENCE OF THE PET FOOD INDUSTRY

Before dogs and cats became domesticated pets, they ranged freely in the wild, eating all sorts of creatures and plants— whatever they could find and catch, including one another. And even today, if you've got a dog or a cat that spends any time at all outside your home, you probably know that he or she loves nothing more than chasing down, catching, and sometimes consuming other animals.

When left to their own devices, dogs and cats have millions of years of genetic heritage that tells them exactly what food is best for them to eat and how to catch and consume it. This food has traditionally been very real—and quite raw.

After dogs and cats became domesticated and began to spend more time in the home than outside it, they most often ate whatever food scraps their humans tossed their way— often meat, organs, fat, or bones, and sometimes raw, sometimes cooked into a stew with bread and other ingredients. While not as common as it was centuries ago, a tradesman known as a knacker or knackerman was responsible for removing animal carcasses from roads, farms, or other places and then processing them into a variety of different products such as grease, glue, bonemeal, animal feed, and more. Basically, dogs and cats ate what we ate, sometimes supplemented with feed derived from processed animal carcasses and whatever creatures they could catch in or out of the home.

This all changed when, in 1860, an American lightning-rod salesman, James Spratt, created one of the first commercially produced dog biscuits. This product—dubbed Spratt's Patent Meat Fibrine Dog Cake—was inspired by hardtack biscuits thrown to street dogs by English sailors. The ingredients were somewhat different, however. While baked hardtack biscuits circa 1860 contained just flour, water, and a pinch of salt, Spratt's creation was made from wheat, beetroot, vegetables, and a top-secret ingredient composed of "the dried unsalted gelatinous parts of Prairie Beef," according to an early advertisement for the product.[2] Dogs loved the hardtack biscuits thrown to them by sailors, and they apparently also loved Spratt's creation.

But Spratt's Patent Meat Fibrine Dog Cake wasn't meant for just *any* dog; it was aimed at an upscale clientele—primarily English country gentlemen and caretakers of show dogs. Little wonder, since a fifty-pound bag of the dog cakes was fairly expensive—reportedly equal to a day's wages for a skilled craftsman of the time. Consider the testimony of a happy customer, William J. Dunbar, published in a Spratt's advertisement from 1876:

> I have much pleasure in bearing personal testimony to their suitability and general efficiency for greyhounds, and in adding that my greyhound, Royal Mary, winner at Altcar of last year's Waterloo Plate, was almost entirely trained for all her last year's engagements upon them.[3]

According to the advertisement, the dog cakes "keep dogs in perfect condition without other food, and obviate worms." In addition, the company sold Spratt's Patent Cat Food, which, the advertisement touts, "entirely supersedes the unwholesome practice of feeding on boiled horse flesh; keeps the cat in perfect health." While there may have been other dog biscuits before Spratt's, this invention was the true beginning of the pet food industry—the first time a commercial business produced a convenient, readily available food product that (the company claimed) contained everything a dog or a cat needed to be completely healthy and happy.

Thus began the big lie that the industry has relied on for more than a century.

After the success of Spratt's pet food, other companies innovated their own products to jump on board this profitable bandwagon. In 1908, the F. H. Bennett Biscuit Company introduced a new dry dog biscuit named Maltoid, which contained milk, meat products, and minerals—and was shaped like a bone. In 1911, the Maltoid dog biscuit was renamed Milk-Bone. According to advertisements at the time, "dogs bark for it" and no other food was necessary for your dog besides it.

The first canned dog food—Ken-L Ration, made primarily of horsemeat, which was in ready supply after the end of World War I—was offered to the public in 1922. The product was so successful that, by the mid-1930s, the company was slaughtering a reported fifty thousand horses each year to fill its cans. Canned dog food quickly dominated, gaining a 90 percent share of the market by 1941. However, dry dog food again took over during World War II, when supplies of meat and the metal used to produce cans were redirected to support the war effort.

When in the early 1950s the soap industry switched from making its products primarily from animal fat to synthetic ingredients and plant oils, all of a sudden a lot of animal fat was available for sale cheap. And where do you think much of that excess animal fat ended up? Right—in dog food as the pet food industry bought it up. Increased amounts of animal fats in dog food required the addition of chemical preservatives to keep the fat from quickly going rancid. One commonly used preservative was ethoxyquin, a synthetic antioxidant developed by Monsanto in the 1950s—originally as a rubber stabilizer. While it did a great job of preserving fat in dog food, it also blew out the livers of many dogs that ate it. Although the chemical is rarely added directly to dog food today by manufacturers, it can still end up in it indirectly through the addition of ingredients such as poultry or fish meals that themselves contain ethoxyquin. In that case, you won't see this ingredient listed on a dog food label.

In 1957, Ralston Purina released Purina Dog Chow. The company's cereal division—which developed the company's popular Chex breakfast cereal—worked on the product for three years, using the company's cooking-food extruder equipment to improve its digestibility, texture, and appearance. Within two years after its introduction, Purina Dog Chow became America's bestselling brand of dog food.

By the 1970s, a new pet food category gained in popularity: premium (sometimes known as superpremium). These "gourmet" products, produced by companies such as Nutro, Iams, and Hill's Pet Nutrition, were marketed to devoted pet parents as the highest-quality, most nutritious, and health-iest pet food available. However, since there is no standard for what constitutes a premium pet food product, the only difference it might actually have from a nonpremium product is a significantly higher price.

And over the past couple of decades, interest in feed-ing dogs and cats organic, raw, and grain-free foods has surged—bringing us full circle, back to when these animals were wild and caught their own food. Long story short, it's taken us the better part of 150 years to realize that the best food for our animal companions is not something that comes out of a bag or can—it's the food that they would naturally eat, given the choice.

One of the things that instigated this major shift in pet food consciousness was the massive pet food recall of 2007. In March 2007, the FDA discovered that dogs and cats were dying after eating certain pet foods. The deaths were traced to vegetable proteins imported from China that were con-taminated with melamine—an organic compound used to create such things as plastic, dinnerware, insulation, clean-ing products, and even Formica counters. The material was commonly used in China as an adulterant for raw milk and animal feed to make it appear higher in protein content than was actually the case, and it eventually found its way into dog and cat food.[4]

According to a 2009 FDA FAQ about the recall, more than 150 brands of pet food (mostly dog and cat, representing tens of millions, and perhaps hundreds of millions, of cans, pouches, and bags) were "voluntarily recalled by a number of companies."[5] During this crisis, the phones were ringing off the hook at most every veterinary hospital all across the United States. At Smith Ridge, we braced ourselves for the deluge of expected calls, especially since our client base came from all over the country. But throughout the entire crisis, we received only three inquiries. And one of those wasn't even a client but a local resident that stopped in. This alone shows you the advantage of proper education. In the wake of this recall I was invited to appear on *Oprah* to discuss proper dog and cat nutrition.

So, what exactly is in those bags and cans of dog and cat food anyway?

A PEEK BEHIND THE CURTAIN

Today, there are six major categories of food for dogs and cats:

- Raw (what dogs and cats originally ate in the wild)
- Cooked at home (such as what I was feeding my own dog and cat companions for many decades, along with a diet of raw food)
- Semimoist (those old Gaines-burgers, and other similar packaged food)
- Canned wet (generally contains mostly water—about 60–75 percent)
- Freeze-dried/dehydrated (food that has all the water extracted)
- Kibble dry (mostly produced using cooking-food extruder machinery)

In the United States, every "can of cat food, bag of dog food, or box of dog treats or snacks in your pantry" is regulated by the US Food and Drug Administration. According to the FDA website:

> The Federal Food, Drug, and Cosmetic Act (FFDCA) requires that all animal foods, like human foods, be safe to eat, produced under sanitary conditions, contain no harmful substances, and be truthfully labeled. In addition, canned pet foods must be processed in conformance with the low acid canned food regulations to ensure the pet food is free of viable microorganisms.

So, how does the FDA know whether something is safe for your animal companion to eat? Actually, there's a law for that. Buried deep within the Code of Federal Regulations (Title 21, chapter 1, subchapter E), the government provides guidance for what exactly can and can't go into animal food. Pet food manufacturers are required to follow these regulations for any products they sell in this country.

Let's say you've decided to start up your own brand of dog food. What ingredients are you allowed to use? According to the government regulations, any substance you put inside your cans must be safe "based only on the views of experts qualified by scientific training and experience to evaluate the safety of substances directly or indirectly added to food." The government provides just two routes for such expert views to be accepted:

- Scientific procedures
- In the case of a substance used in food prior to January 1, 1958, through experience based on common use in food[6]

That's all well and good, but now we're back to the original question: What ingredients are you allowed to put into that dog food you're planning to start manufacturing and selling? Glad you asked. The use of beef, chicken, duck, bison, fish, and most any animal is fine—they have commonly been used as food for eons. However, the government also says that meat by-products, poultry by-products, meat meal and bonemeal, and animal fats are okay, too.[7] So, too, fruits and vegetables, grains, and other whole foods.

But what about all those additives that you see on the side of many bags and cans of pet food? Buried deep within the Code of Federal Regulations (Title 21, chapter 1, subchapter E, part 582) is a list of substances that are "generally recognized as safe" (GRAS) for their intended use in animal food and drinking water. This long laundry list of items considered to be safe by the US government includes:

- Spices and other natural seasonings and flavorings—everything from alfalfa seed to horseradish to vanilla
- Essential oils, oleoresins (solvent-free), and natural extractives (including distillates)—such things as curaçao orange peel, hops, and peppermint
- Natural substances and extractives (solvent-free) used in conjunction with spices and other natural seasonings and flavorings—including brown algae, cognac oil, and musk
- Synthetic flavoring substances and adjuvants—such things

as acetaldehyde, 3-methyl-3-phenyl glycidic acid ethyl ester, and glycerol
- Trace minerals added to animal feeds—from cobalt to iodine to zinc
- General-purpose food additives—including hydrochloric acid, helium, propane, and many more[8]

Ironically, the federal government's list of substances prohibited from use in animal food is quite a bit shorter. Here you go:

- Gentian violet
- Propylene glycol in or on cat food
- Protein in ruminant feed derived from mammalian tissues (with a number of exceptions)
- Materials derived from cattle with bovine spongiform encephalopathy (BSE)—again, with a number of exceptions)[9]

That's it.

But there's more to what's inside that can or bag of dog or cat food than just what the FDA says can go in there. One more organization has a lot to say about it: the Association of American Feed Control Officials (AAFCO), which was founded in 1909. While the organization has no direct regulatory authority over pet food—it has no enforcement power—it has had a tremendous influence over it. According to the AAFCO website:

AAFCO's longstanding purpose has been to serve as a venue for feed regulators to explore the problems encountered in administering feed laws; to develop just and equitable standards, definitions and policies for the enforcement of feed laws; and to promote uniformity in laws, regulations and enforcement policies. AAFCO has created a large number of models providing guidance, definitions, terms and best-management practices in addition to the Model Bill and Model Feed Regulations (including Model Pet Food Regulations).[10]

AAFCO sets the standards for what ingredients should and shouldn't go into pet food and animal feed—including the definition of *complete and balanced*—package labeling, and more. According to AAFCO, pet food is *complete* when "the product contains all the nutrients required," and *balanced* when "the nutrients are present in the correct ratios."[11] We'll take a closer look at AAFCO's definitions in the next section.

Regardless of which dog or cat food you choose, you should handle it carefully to avoid contamination and illness—just as you would handle food for your family and yourself. Here's some handling advice from the UK Pet Food Manufacturers' Association:

- Only buy products that are in good condition. You should see no visible signs of damage to the packaging such as dents, tears, discolorations, etc.
- Wash your hands with hot water and soap after handling either your pet or their food.
- After each use, wash your pet's bowls, dishes, and utensils

with soap and hot water, rinse properly, and dry before the next use.
- Correctly store unsealed containers / open bags to limit any risk of cross contamination.
- When storing pet food in the fridge, ensure raw products are at the bottom. You can find the storage instructions on each package.[12]

It's no big secret that there is a lot of controversy about pet food ingredients, and what is truly healthy for our animal companions—both over the short and long runs. In the next section, we'll take a closer look at this controversy.

ASK DR. MARTY

Q: I'm vegan. Can my dog and cat companions be vegan, too?

A: Cats are obligate carnivores, and almost across the board the answer for them is *no*. Meat is the most necessary ingredient in their diets. And it should be good-quality meat—not low-grade by-products. With dogs, the answer is not so simple. They are considered omnivores, and their digestive systems are quite capable of digesting and deriving nutrients from fruits and vegetables. While they can obtain nutrients from plant matter, these nutrients are more in the categories of vitamins, minerals, and antioxidants—they're missing a number of essential elements that are derived from animal-protein sources. Unless done well, making dogs vegans without expert supervision can lead to some serious health problems, and unfortunately I have witnessed this quite a number of times in clinical practice.

That being said, at the writing of this book, there is a movement to change this—especially because of the tremendously negative impact raising meat for the pet food industry has on the environment of our planet, not to mention the pain and suffering these animals go through as they are raised and eventually brought to slaughter. Other options that could work well include an ancient fungus called koji (*Aspergillus oryzae*)—which is used to ferment soybeans to create soy sauce and miso, and rice to make sake—or insects such as crickets. While crickets are decidedly not vegan, their use as a food source for dogs would help decrease the current dependence on the use of mammals, poultry, and fish as major ingredients in pet food. These and other food sources have the potential to satisfy many if not all of the nutritional requirements for dogs living healthy lives.

If and when this can happen and is proven effective in long-term studies, I am certainly all for it and uphold the old biblical statement "The wolf also shall dwell with the lamb, and the leopard shall lie down with the kid."

THE PROBLEM WITH DOG AND CAT FOOD

Remember AAFCO—the organization that sets the standards for what goes into pet food? As people have become more enlightened as to what constitutes the healthiest diet for their animal companions, AAFCO's standards have come under increasing scrutiny. Dr. Ian Billinghurst is a longtime critic of AAFCO and the commercial pet food industry, and a proponent of raw food diets. He originated the BARF (biologically appropriate raw food) diet, which according to Dr. Billinghurst "is about feeding dogs and cats the diet they evolved to eat over millions of years of genetic adaptation."

I met Dr. Billinghurst for the first time when I was invited to be a keynote speaker for a raw-pet-food company—Carnivora, in Saskatoon, Saskatchewan—which sells tons of raw meat each month all across Canada. The event was held over the weekend, and there were two other keynote speakers: my friend Dr. Rob Silver, who is an expert on the use of nutraceuticals, cannabis, and CBD oil with dogs and cats, and Dr. Billinghurst. I've known Rob for almost forty years, but I had not yet crossed paths with Dr. Billinghurst.

Although I was pretty booked up with my own presentations—I spoke for several hours on Saturday and Sunday—I made a point of listening to Dr. Billinghurst speak. I was blown away. He explained how cancer is the expression of a preexisting genetic program of ceaseless reproduction developed and used by our single-celled ancestors 2 billion years ago. After explaining why cancer exists, he explained what to do about it: go back to nature, feeding our animal companions healthy, raw food that is species appropriate.

According to Dr. Billinghurst, it can clearly be shown that 90 to 95 percent of dogs diagnosed each year with all sorts of diseases and physical and mental problems—including cancer, autoimmune diseases, allergies, renal failure, and many more—actually developed their diseases while eating foods that met the standards set by AAFCO.[13] Dogs and cats have adverse reactions to food, says Dr. Billinghurst, because of the widespread use of "fake food, industrial food, cooked and processed grain-based pet food, a group of products [that], as a profession, we veterinarians endorse, trust, promote, sell, and actively defend on a daily basis."[14]

The heart of the BARF diet is whole, healthy, raw food that "mimics the diet of a wild or feral animal"—including meat, bones, organ meats, vegetables, fruits, and so on. Says Dr. Billinghurst, "You can enhance the diet you produce with healthy supplements such as vitamins, essential fatty acids, probiotics, kelp, alfalfa powder, various herbs, etc."[15] You definitely won't find commercially produced food—dry or wet—in the BARF diet.

Dry pet food became so popular for some good reasons. It had great shelf life, was easy to store, wasn't as heavy as cans of wet food, and was less expensive because combinations of cheap, low-grade cereal grains (corn, wheat, barley, rice, and so forth) were used as key ingredients. Sometimes it's not even the whole grains that make it into dog and cat food—it's the floor sweepings or waste by-products (also known as middlings or mill run) from the production of human food. The big companies that produced the food created a false foundation of science—often backed by veterinary professionals—to support their claims that it was healthier for our animal companions, and we bought it.

In just one example, some of these companies claimed that corn is the most digestible and usable source of protein for dogs, which is just ridiculous. What's more likely is that the companies put corn in the bags because it was the cheapest grain that year, then they wrote a story about how great corn is for your dog. If barley is cheaper than corn the next year, then they'll write a new story about barley being the new "wonder food" for dogs. A lot of this is just marketing.

How did we come to accept the story we were told by the pet food industry? Because they (supposedly) conducted lots of research, and they (definitely) produced lots of statistics (and advertising) that loudly trumpeted their claims. Independent research, however, shows that much pet food is not nearly as nutritious as its manufacturers would have us believe.

In an online article, Dr. Karen Becker explains that "about 95 percent of dry pet diets are manufactured using the extrusion process"—where mixes of wet and dry ingredients are cooked at high temperatures and, under high pressure, extruded or pushed through shaped die plates, cut, dried, then packaged. According to Dr. Becker, research shows that this process removes much of the nutrition from the resulting food, including vitamin loss and protein denaturation resulting in the reduction of available amino acids. Says Dr. Becker, "In my opinion, the reduction in amino acids could be one of the main reasons we are seeing more heart disease, including dilated cardiomyopathy (DCM), in many companion animals today."[16]

Dr. Becker cites a June 27, 2019, update by the FDA on its investigation into the rash of DCM cases. According to the FDA update, the number of reports of DCM in dogs and cats submitted to the agency jumped from just 1 in 2014 to 320 in 2018. (Note: Some of the reports submitted to the

FDA included more than one affected animal.) In the first four months of 2019—through April 30—197 reports of DCM in dogs and cats were submitted to the agency. According to the FDA, of the 515 reports of DCM in dogs it received between January 1, 2014, and April 30, 2019—representing a total of 560 affected dogs—452 (88 percent) of the reports involved dogs that were fed a diet of dry kibble.[17] That's a smoking gun if I've ever seen one, and it's a good reason to reconsider your dog's diet if she is eating kibble—especially if your dog is a large breed most prone to DCM.

Back in the 1980s, cats went through a similar DCM epidemic. According to scientists at the University of California, Davis, tens of thousands of cats were dying each year from DCM. The cause was traced to a deficiency of the amino acid taurine in dry cat food. Taurine regulates the entry of calcium into heart tissue—required for the heart to beat. When a dog or cat gets DCM, its heart can no longer pump blood through its body, and without proper treatment death usually follows within just days or weeks.

Surprisingly, cats can't synthesize taurine, but most other mammals—including dogs—can, if they're healthy. So, cats need to eat animal protein or take supplements to get the taurine they need. After the source of the cat DCM epidemic was identified, cat food manufacturers dramatically increased the amount of taurine in their products by law and the disease became more controlled.

The current rash of dog DCM cases has been tied by some to the consumption of grain-free diets. I don't believe that the issue is whether grain is present in food—ultimately, it's the presence or absence of animal tissue. Nothing in grains supports heart health in carnivores. When food man-ufacturers replace animal protein with plant-based protein or carbohydrates, regardless of their source, the amount of taurine will naturally decline.

One theory suggests that grain substitutes such as peas, lentils, legumes, and potatoes contain proteins called lectins, which block the absorption or utilization of taurine from the intestine. Another theory is that these substitutes contain dangerous molds that produce mycotoxins that are damaging to the dogs' hearts. And lastly, it is now evident in animal studies that glyphosate damages the heart, and these grain substitutes are glyphosate carriers.[18] And when this food is manufactured using the high-heat, high-pressure extrusion process—as most dry kibble is, denaturing what relatively small amounts of amino acids were in there—then you've got a recipe for disaster.

You've got a recipe for DCM.

NUTRITION—IT'S ABSURDLY SIMPLE

BY DR. IAN BILLINGHURST

What should we feed our dogs and cats to ensure normal growth, a long life, and maximum freedom from disease? Do we follow the complex AAFCO rules, or do we feed those foods animals have evolved to require? Today, even the most ardent advocates of *raw* (biologically appropriate) food for dogs and cats complicate matters by attempting to follow AAFCO guidelines. Yet, such rules apply only to processed pet foods. This AAFCO approach, as taken by today's (highly credentialed) veterinary nutritionists, attempts to design pet foods based on our limited knowledge of nutrient requirements, and using (often toxic) highly denatured, nutritionally impoverished waste materials. These nutrition professionals actually fear real food. Their nutrient-centered approach produces the cooked and processed products that support a vet's bottom line.

The results of feeding these products fill our veterinary waiting rooms and hospitals, not exactly what we want for our dogs and cats. This does not have to be because formulating a healthy nutritional program is absurdly simple, so long as you follow evolutionary principles. Our cats and dogs did not evolve eating processed pet foods. To be truly healthy, we must free our cats and dogs from the nutritionally incompetent products designed by veterinary nutritionists and feed them the food they have been eating for millions of years.

Yes, it is that simple.

We must look after our furry family members the way we look after our cars, where we only ever use the fuel, lubrication, spare parts, and maintenance schedule specified by the manufacturer. Evolution is the process that manufactured our cats and dogs; therefore, their bodies require a nutritional program based on the broad range and balance of the actual foods, *raw* and *whole*, they evolved eating. This food-centered approach to nutrition (rather than being nutrient centered) supplies all essential nutrients, in perfect balance, including those nutrients that nutritional science does not (as yet) know about or does not as yet understand as necessary for optimum health! When properly formulated, an evolutionary program of nutrition is both legally and, more important, biologically complete and balanced.

To produce this diet, simply ensure the food matches (in form and proportion) the body parts found in small mammals, birds, fish, insects, or reptiles (preferably all five), together with other healthy foods such as yogurt, natural oils, eggs, low-glycemic veggies (crushed and raw), kelp, herbs, etc. These additional foods mimic the gut contents (including feces) that dogs (and to a lesser extent cats) have eaten over evolutionary time.

There you have it. And rather than each meal, it is the overall nutritional program that must be complete and balanced, just as it has always been. For our dogs, we include extra bones (dogs are more scavenging than cats) and more vegetable material (dogs are more omnivorous than cats). Such a nutritional program will meet both species' entire nutritional requirements. Nutrition . . . it's absurdly simple!

For more information, please visit www.drianbillinghurst .com.

CAN A HEALTHIER GUT MEAN A HAPPIER DOG?

Gut health seems to be the new frontier in medicine. Studies demonstrate correlations between behavior and the microbiome in toddlers, mice, chimpanzees, and now dogs. So, can a healthier gut mean a happier dog? You bet it can! Let's consider the answers to three specific questions:

1. How or why does the microbiome impact a dog's overall health?

There's an old saying, "You are what you eat!" I don't quite agree with that. As vital as good food is, I feel a better adage would be "You are what you absorb and metabolize!" The same thing applies to our canine companions. Put high-quality gasoline into a car that is out of tune and the car is not going to perform well. As important as a high-quality, species-appropriate diet is for our animal companions, without a proper and healthy microbiome, that good food is not going to be properly digested and broken down, which then shortchanges metabolism.

2. Can a dog's stomach affect his behavior?

Absolutely! We are all well aware of how food leftovers that sit in a garbage pail tend to rot, ferment, and stink even after as little as a day. Without a healthy, functioning microbiome to properly and fully digest foods in the gut, a similar process occurs—leading to the absorption of these stinking fermentation substances that not only have a negative effect on health, but also on mood and behavior. And even more important, the neurotransmitter substance serotonin (commonly called the "Don't worry, be happy" biochemical messenger of the brain) is mostly produced in the gut. Improper gut health leads to low levels of serotonin production, which has a direct, negative effect on a dog's behavior. Are there ways to treat imbalanced gut health that might impact a dog's happiness? Yes! By simply supplementing a dog's diet with a high-quality probiotic, prebiotic, and even digestive-enzyme supplement, science has demonstrated this has a positive effect on serotonin production.

3. Based on the research or clients in your own practice, have you witnessed a dog's behavior improve—maybe less fear or less stress—when gut health was restored?

Without exaggeration, thousands of times over my forty-five-plus-year career as a practicing veterinarian specializing in healthy diet and supplementation. Not only do so many of my canine patients become more active and appear to be happier with less anger and aggressiveness, one of the most common things I have heard is "She found and played with her ball or toy for the first time in years!"

ASK DR. MARTY

Q: Are there any human foods that I should avoid feeding our family dog? He seems to love to eat everything!

A: Most definitely! Just because a particular food is healthy for you to eat doesn't mean that it's equally healthy for the dogs in your life. Here are eight foods that are okay for humans, but potentially harmful for dogs:

1. AVOCADO

This green goddess of a fruit has gotten a lot of attention in the human health and wellness world for its high content of healthy fats, including the essential omega fatty acid oleic acid. However, avocados also contain a phytochemical called persin. If eaten in fairly large amounts, it can potentially be harmful to dogs. Not only that, but the essential fatty acids found in avocado, if ingested, may cause your pup to suffer from a variety of problems, including upset stomach, pancreatitis, shortness of breath, and even a buildup of fluids in the chest.

2. COFFEE

While your dog might enjoy sitting next to you while you eat breakfast, don't pour an extra cup of coffee for the occasion. Coffee contains methylated xanthine, which stimulates the nervous system. Dogs who consume coffee may experience a disruption in their nervous system—leading to anxiety, restlessness, heart palpitations, vomiting, and even death.

3. GRAPES AND RAISINS

When my first book was published in 1999, I wrote about how I would throw grapes to my dogs as snacks. However, at about the time I was writing that book, researchers started to become aware that grapes were toxic to dogs. As the internet emerged, and Google made searching for information reliable, fast, and easy, the public started to become aware of this potential danger. To date, I have

still not witnessed nor come across even one incident of grape toxicity in dogs, but it does seem to be the case. The biological mechanism for why this happens is still not yet understood. Could it be the chemicals sprayed on some grapes before harvest? Perhaps. So, to be on the safe side, do not feed your animal companions grapes or raisins, but also don't live in fear of this pending disaster.

4. CHOCOLATE

Chocolate is derived from the seeds of *Theobroma cacao*—a plant used for centuries by humans as a medicine due to active chemical constituents known to boost immunity against common infections, among other things. However, one of the most notable compounds in chocolate—theobromine—has been associated with toxicity in pets at a dose of a 250-gram packet of cocoa powder (approximately 8.8 ounces) or half of a 250-gram block of cooking chocolate.[19] I found it becomes toxic at 40–50 mg/kg, which is approximately 20 mg per pound.

5. MACADAMIA NUTS

These fatty nuts are native to Australia, and their delicious flavor is wonderful. Alas, dogs should absolutely never eat them. Studies have shown that, even in small amounts, macadamia nuts can be toxic to dogs, leading to motor difficulties, weakness, difficulty breathing, tremors, and swollen limbs. The toxic dose for dogs ranges from 2.4–62.4 grams per kilogram (2.2 pounds) body weight.[20]

6. XYLITOL

Xylitol is an artificial sweetener found in candy, sugar-free chewing gum, toothpaste, baked goods, and other "diet" human foods. Studies show that consuming xylitol can cause a significant, and often sustained, insulin-mediated hypoglycemic crisis in dogs. This sudden drop in blood sugar may cause depression, ataxia, seizures, or collapse in dogs, and potentially more serious problems, including liver damage and even death.[21]

7. ALCOHOL

Your dog is your best friend, and that may make you think that when you have an alcoholic beverage, the dog might also want a sip. But alcoholic beverages can be toxic to dogs, as they cannot tolerate alcohol, even in small amounts. So do not give your dog any type of alcohol, including beer, liquor, or even mouthwash, as it has been linked to toxicosis in dogs. This also includes fermented vegetables, as they contain small amounts of ethanol alcohol.[22]

8. MILK AND ICE CREAM

If your dogs had the same stomach as you do, these foods wouldn't cause them any problem. However, because they don't have the necessary enzymes inside their gastrointestinal tract to break down cow milk, eating it (in any form except, perhaps, fermented, such as yogurt) can cause mild to severe cases of digestive upset including diarrhea, and vomiting. In short, dogs are lactose intolerant (just like some humans). So, the next time you're thinking of giving your animal companion a Puppuccino whipped cream treat at Starbucks, don't give in. It's for her own good.

TIME TO GET REAL

What should you feed your animal companions for best health? Aim for the ideal. And that's the big word: *aim*. Diet decisions are not a matter of right or wrong. If you understand what is ideal, you can then create a feeding program that will help move your pet closer to the healthiest diet options. In general, the more real food your dogs and cats eat, the healthier they will be.

The list below outlines how our feeding choices for our pets (companion carnivores) can affect their health. The closer to the upper-level choices, the better the chance for optimal health. Many of you may likely be in the middle ranges most of the time. That is fine, as long as you always press toward the ideal.

1. Hunted, raw prey (not realistic in modern society).
2. Fresh, raw meats (including freeze-dried raw meats), bones, organ meats with small amounts of fresh vegetables. Include a well-rounded vitamin/mineral mix and omega-3 essential fatty acids. You can prepare your own raw diet using meat/bone pieces and parts, or you can use prepared ground products.
3. Fresh-cooked meats and organs, with small amounts of fresh vegetables. Include a vitamin/mineral mix consist-

brown rice. When we adopted him, he was emaciated from eating horrible, low-grade food at the dog-racing track. This is why we still feed him home-cooked food. Approximately 40 percent of his diet is cooked chicken with brown rice, and the rest is raw. That's perfect for him.

Our other dog companions, Tilly and Joey, are getting 85 percent raw or freeze-dried raw—they have been eating raw food from puppyhood. Most of our cat companions are eating 100 percent raw, but we also give them some healthy, single-ingredient canned food, too. Why? Because they love it.

Food allergies are also a big concern, and you can make a difference in the life of your animal companions with the diet choices you make for them. We do a lot of food-allergy testing in our clinic, based on a blood sample. The results aren't 100 percent accurate, but we've learned so much. I believe that the most accurate way to tell if your pet has a food allergy is through a process of trial and error using what's known as an elimination diet. In this diet you put a dog or a cat on a strict, single-protein diet for a time, see how the pet does, then switch to another protein and start over. We'll take a closer look at that in chapter 7.

THE SALMONELLA CONUNDRUM

I must address one more thing in the final section of this chapter, a topic that causes a lot of confusion: salmonella. We all know that salmonella infections (salmonellosis) can and do wreak havoc on humans—according to the Centers for Disease Control and Prevention (CDC), an estimated 1.2 million cases are reported in the United States each year—leading to 23,000 hospitalizations and 450 deaths—with 94 percent of those cases transmitted by food. Symptoms of salmonellosis include diarrhea, abdominal cramps, fever, and occasionally nausea and vomiting.[23] Given the legitimate concerns about salmonella infections and humans, should we be equally concerned about salmonella and our animal companions?

Maybe not.

In September 2019, the CDC issued an Investigation Notice regarding an outbreak of multidrug-resistant salmonella infections linked to contact with pig-ear dog treats. According to the notice, 143 salmonella infections in thirty-five states have been related to pig-ear dog treats.[24] But notice one thing: these were infections in humans, not dogs. The CDC notice was not out of concern for dogs, but because humans handling pig-ear dog treats were getting sick from them.

The *Salmonella* bacterium is quite common in the wild and can be found in the digestive tracts of many different kinds of animals, including reptiles, rodents, birds and poultry, horses, cows, pigs—and dogs and cats.

Which brings us back to the question: Should we be concerned about salmonella and our animal companions? Based on the evidence, I would say the answer is no. Salmonella is more of an issue of hygiene than of disease. Think, for example, about the threat of salmonella in your home from the raw chicken from your supermarket as you prepare it for your family for dinner. I'm certain you take every precaution to ensure that you don't get *Salmonella* bacteria all over your kitchen. You wash your hands, you cut the chicken on a nonporous cutting board, you wash well every surface that came in contact with the chicken, you thoroughly clean your utensils, and so forth. Handled properly, you can safely introduce raw chicken into your home and live to tell the tale.

While the *Salmonella* organism naturally inhabits the gastrointestinal tract of many dogs and cats, its presence is at a subclinical level—that is, the dogs and cats don't become ill as a result. According to the *Merck Veterinary Manual*—the bible of veterinary medicine:

> Many dogs and cats are asymptomatic carriers of salmonellae. Clinical disease is uncommon, but when it is seen, it is often associated with hospitalization, another infection or debilitating condition in adults, or exposure to large numbers of the bacteria in puppies and kittens, in which enteritis may be common.[25]

So, while I would not intentionally feed any dog or cat food that I knew was teaming with *Salmonella* (in that case it would probably be rotten and should be discarded anyway), I would not worry about exposing my dogs or cats to salmonella when feeding them a normal diet—whether raw or not.

THERE'S BEEN A SPIKE IN CANINE HEART DISEASE—WHAT CAN YOU DO?

by Dr. Karen Becker

It's no big secret that we veterinarians have seen a sudden rash of cases of nutritionally related dilated cardiomyopathy (DCM, a type of heart disease) in dogs. The current evidence appears to link grain-free kibble and taurine deficiency with the mini-epidemic.

Here are the facts from a recent FDA update on diet-related canine DCM:

- Between January 1, 2014, and April 30, 2019, there were reports of 560 affected dogs and 119 deaths.
- The number of reported cases (which also included a small number of cats) jumped from 3 in 2017 to 320 in 2018, and was already at 197 through April 30, 2019.
- Golden retrievers, mixed breeds, and Labrador retrievers were the breeds most frequently reported.
- The vast majority of affected dogs were fed a dry food (kibble) diet.
- Of the diets, 91 percent were grain-free and 93 percent contained peas and/or lentils.
- The most common proteins in the diets were chicken, lamb, and fish.

It's important to note that some in both the veterinary community and the pet food industry have campaigned to lay the blame on "BEG" (boutique, exotic, grain-free) diets. Some of these folks imply or actually recommend that pet parents switch to a big name-brand, grain-based dog food containing a nonexotic protein source. However, the FDA report exonerates both dog food found in pet food boutiques (the *B* in *BEG*), and exotic protein sources (the *E*).

Many of the diets fed to the dogs who developed nutritionally related DCM were about as far from "boutique" brands as it gets, including formulas produced by the biggest pet food companies in the United States: Mars Petcare / Royal Canin (which owns Nutro, California Natural, and Evo), Nestlé Purina PetCare (Merrick), Hill's Pet Nutrition, Smucker (Rachael Ray and Natural Balance), and General Mills / Blue Buffalo.

In addition, as noted in the data points above, the most common proteins in the diets were chicken, lamb, and fish, none of which are considered exotic. Sadly, despite the FDA's clear evidence to the contrary, the "experts" continue to insist part of the problem is exotic protein sources.

What we have left after debunking the myth that boutique brands and exotic proteins are the problem is the *G* in *BEG*—grain-free—and, indeed, the vast majority of the diets the dogs were fed were grain-free kibble.

DCM has multiple causes. Genetics and nutrition both play a role, and the nutrition component also has many causes. For example, the lectins and other antinutrients in grain-free kibble may be contributors. In addition, toxic levels of metals (iron, copper, and cobalt) have been linked to DCM in humans. However, the elephant in the room is protein deficiency, which when coupled with high levels of certain minerals causes DCM in humans that is reversible with added protein in the diet.

All pet food contains three sources of calories and nutrients: fat, protein, and carbohydrates, which occur in varying amounts depending on the formula. The amount of each of these components means the difference between health and disease and also defines how species appropriate the food is. Pet foods become protein deficient because of four main reasons:

- Excessive carbohydrates
- Excessive fat
- Processing methods
- Poor-quality raw ingredients and synthetic add-ins

Bottom line: The answer to DCM isn't to add grains back into grain-free formulas, nor is it to add synthetic amino acids into basically vegan pet foods. The answer is to feed an abundance of biologically appropriate, real meat as the foundation of any nutritionally optimized formula or recipe.

So, what can you do to provide your furry friends with the healthiest diet possible? The following to-do list is designed to help you be self-sufficient when choosing how to best nourish your animal companions.

Step 1—Calculate the macronutrients in your pet's food. Find the guaranteed analysis on your pet food label. Carbohydrates should not exceed 20 percent for any dog or cat food without concern for meat-based amino acid deficiencies occurring over time. A dog's ancestral diet supplies approximately 50 percent of calories from fat and 50 percent of calories from protein (lean, human-grade, fresh meat).

Step 2—Rotate through a variety of foods, brands, and proteins. Rotating flavors within just one brand of foods means that if there's excessive cobalt or iron, your pet is probably still at risk. All meats have a different amino acid profile, so providing a variety of proteins offers your dog nutritional diversity. If you feed your dog a home-made diet, follow a recipe you know meets minimum nutrient requirements and uses only 85 percent lean meats. Guessing gets people into trouble, and rotation over time statistically doesn't work. Feed frozen diets within three months of preparation or manufacturing.

Step 3—Add amino-rich toppers and treats to a well-balanced, diversified diet. The key to avoiding DCM, a deficiency-induced disease, is to offer a variety of well-formulated, commercially available fresh-food diets or to prepare nutritionally optimized meals yourself. Seafood is especially high in taurine and other amino acids, as are animal hearts. An easy way to supply additional amino acids to your pet's meals is to divvy up a can of sardines (packed in water) per thirty pounds of dog over a week. (So, if you have a sixty-pound dog, spread out two cans over a week, and so on.)

Step 4—Have your veterinarian check your dog's taurine levels if you have a predisposed breed. Ask your vet to submit both plasma and serum taurine levels directly to the UC Davis Veterinary Medicine Amino Acid Laboratory. If you don't know your pet's breed, do a DNA test, so you can determine if your dog may have a genetic predisposition you didn't know about.

Step 5—Provide supplementation if your dog tests low for taurine. If your dog has low blood taurine levels, the first step is to change the diet. As I mentioned, I don't recommend supplementing a nutritionally inadequate diet. I recommend rotating through a variety of better-quality, meat-based foods and supplementing simultaneously with taurine-rich foods, as well as:

- **Taurine.** Talk with your veterinarian about starting supplementation at 500 mg for every twenty-five pounds of body weight twice daily.
- **Ubiquinol.** This reduced form of CoQ_{10} is beneficial in supporting at-risk animals, with no side effects. Talk with your veterinarian about starting with 1 mg per pound of body weight one to two times daily.
- **L-carnitine.** Talk with your vet about starting supplementation with L-carnitine at 500 mg for every twenty-five pounds of body weight twice daily.

Step 6—Schedule an annual wellness exam. Include a CardioPet proBNP heart health test for predisposed breeds. After six years of age, I recommend a complete physical twice a year.

Thank you, Dr. Becker. Here's my two cents on canine heart disease: Nothing in grain supports carnivore heart health, so please don't be fooled by these fear-based stories that go viral on the internet. Also, I am just waiting for studies that show the potential link between GMOs—and especially glyphosate—and damage to heart function, as they are found in high levels in the foods used to substitute for grain.

ASK DR. MARTY

Q: I've noticed that there seems to be a big upsurge of interest in freeze-dried raw diets for pets. How do you compare these with good old traditional raw diets?

A: Great question! It would appear that feeding an all-raw diet to our carnivore companions would best simulate nature and any processing would diminish nutritional value, right? As much as I would love to see a raw diet available to the masses, the expense of refrigerated shipping would make it far too expensive for most people. And then you have the issue of live pathogens—just one contaminated package could shut down the production line for a long time. Freeze-drying removes just the moisture while retaining all the original nutritive value. With no moisture, bacteria and enzyme degradation stops, and the food stays stable for long periods without refrigeration. Extracting the moisture also diminishes the food's weight tremendously, cutting shipping costs. So, having a food such as this would go along with my desire to help dogs and cats globally, and not just in my own practice.

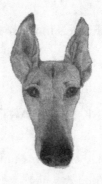

5

THE TREMENDOUS POWER OF NUTRACEUTICALS

There were never so many able, active
minds at work on the problems
of diseases as now, and all their discoveries
are tending to the simple truth—
that you can't improve on nature.
—THOMAS EDISON

Within the universe of pet nutrition, one trend in particular stands out: nutraceuticals. According to Stephen DeFelice, who coined the term, a *nutraceutical* is simply "food or part of a food that provides medical or health benefits, including the prevention and treatment of disease." As you have likely already guessed, the term is a mash-up of the words *nutrition* and *pharmaceutical.* In the case of humans, this can mean anything from Quaker Oats—which contain antioxidants and soluble fiber that its manufacturer claims can lower cholesterol levels—to dietary supplements such as vitamins, minerals, herbs, and amino acids.

But do nutraceuticals such as these have the same kind of positive effect on our animal companions as they do on us humans? In my experience, the answer is clearly *yes*. However, it's taken many years for the veterinary establishment to come around to this way of thinking. As I mentioned in chapter 3, in 1978, I heard that a group of conventional veterinarians were making noise that my license should be suspended because I dared to recommend giving dogs a glucosamine sulfate supplement to treat their arthritis.

I remember when, back in the early nineties, the FDA decided to start raiding health food stores to crack down on the claims of manufacturers of vitamins and other nutraceuticals. A *New York Times* article from August 1992 described a series of raids on Texas health food stores—including Whole Foods Markets and Sun Harvest Farms—to confiscate a variety of food supplements:

> In Texas, state health inspectors raided health food stores across the state in May and, as startled customers and bystanders watched in amazement, removed hundreds of products, including vitamin C, aloe vera products, and herbal teas.[1]

That was then, but this is now.

Today, one-third of all US households with dogs use supplements—including many millions of dollars' worth of glucosamine each year—along with one-fifth of all US households with cats.[2] This sea change in practice occurred over four decades.

Before we go any further, let's first consider the differences, if any, between what we call supplements and nutraceuticals.

Supplements—more specifically, *dietary supplements*—have been around for ages. They include a remarkably broad collection of things meant to supplement the human diet (or, for our purposes, the diets of our animal companions). For decades, the US federal government tried to regulate supplements—fighting the supplement industry, which was concerned that the government would shut them down. In 1994, Congress finally passed the Dietary Supplement Health and Education Act, which, among other things, defined what a supplement is, set labeling requirements, and created a system of regulatory review by the FDA.

When he signed the act in October 1994, President Bill Clinton said, "After several years of intense efforts, manufacturers, experts in nutrition, and legislators, acting in a conscientious alliance with consumers at the grassroots level, have moved successfully to bring common sense to the treatment of dietary supplements under regulation and law."[3]

Notably, the act does not require supplement manufacturers to prove the safety of supplements before they can be sold. The FDA can step in and ban a supplement only when it is proven to be harmful or dangerous. Also, keep in mind that the FDA has determined that the law does not apply to animal food, including pet food. "Thus," says the FDA, "there is no 'dietary supplement' regulatory classification for animal food substances and products. They are considered either 'foods' or 'new animal drugs' depending on the intended use.[4]

According to section 3 of the Dietary Supplement Health and Education Act, a dietary supplement is defined as a product (other than tobacco) intended to supplement the diet that contains one or more of the following dietary ingredients:

A. A vitamin
B. A mineral
C. An herb or other botanical
D. An amino acid
E. A substance used to increase the total dietary intake
F. A concentrate, metabolite, constituent, extract, or combination of any ingredients described in clause A, B, C, D, or E[5]

So, most anything that you might yourself take as a supplement to your normal diet is covered by this definition. Do you take a daily multivitamin? That's a supplement. Omega-3 or fish oil capsules? That's a supplement. A meal-replacement drink such as Ensure or SlimFast? That's a supplement.

So, what then is a *nutraceutical* and what makes it different from a supplement?

In my mind and my veterinary practice, there's no difference between a dietary supplement and a nutraceutical. *Nutraceutical* is just a more modern term for *supplement,* in much the same way that today we most often use the term *integrative* instead of *holistic.* They both mean the same thing.

So, for the most part, I use the term *nutraceutical* instead of *supplement* in this book.

You should know that AAFCO, the Association of American Feed Control Officials, which sets the nutrient standards for dogs and cats, is on record as being against the use of many dietary supplements. According to the AAFCO website, "The first question a pet owner should consider about supplements is whether a pet really needs them in the first place. Generally speaking, healthy dogs and cats that are fed a complete and balanced diet appropriate for their life stage do not."[6]

I so strongly disagree with this.

While this position would make sense if the food people gave to their animal companions was as nutritious as the unadulterated food that their ancestors readily obtained in the wild thousands of years ago, this is clearly not the case today. We do the dogs and the cats in our lives a great disservice by not providing them with all the nutrition—including nutraceuticals, as necessary—required to maintain good health.

WHY NUTRACEUTICALS?

Now that you know what a nutraceutical is, that leaves a couple of burning questions: Why add them to your animal companion's diet? If you feed your animal friend a well-balanced diet in accordance with AAFCO guidelines, shouldn't that be enough?

Nutraceuticals have a definite place in the diet of any animal, whether human or your favorite dog or cat. The soil in which we grow our crops has been seriously degraded over time. In its report titled *The Status of the World's Soil Resources*, the Food and Agriculture Organization of the United Nations noted:

> The overwhelming conclusion of the report is that the majority of the world's soil resources are in only fair, poor, or very poor condition and that conditions are getting worse in far more cases than they are improving. In particular, 33 percent of land is moderately to highly degraded due to erosion, salinization, compaction, acidification, and chemical pollution of soils.[7]

The nutritionally deficient crops grown in these degraded soils are then fed to animals—cows, chickens, pigs, and so on—that are used in pet food. And I'm not even talking about the scourge of glyphosate, the weed killer linked to cancer that has found its way into many food sources. Nutraceuticals are necessary to make up for the deficiencies we humans have created in the earth and in the food chain that is derived from it. Nutraceuticals should truly be used to supplement the diet—they act indirectly on the patient through what he or she eats.

Thousands of years ago, I imagine that the ancestors of today's domestic dogs and cats had little if any degenerative disease or cancer. Millennia ago, the earth had not yet been degraded by humans, and everything animals ate was at its peak nutrition. A rabbit ate plants that grew in soil that was fertile, rich, and filled with nutrients. When a wolf or wildcat hunted down and ate the rabbit, it gained the benefit of all that nutrition. As the old saying goes, let thy food be thy medicine.

Today, that is no longer the case, despite (and, I believe, in many cases because of) mankind's efforts to boost crop yields. An analysis of data prepared by government scientists in Canada from 1951 through 1999 revealed that vitamin A levels in potatoes declined 100 percent, vitamin C and iron declined 57 percent, and calcium declined 28 percent. In addition, levels of riboflavin declined 50 percent and thiamine 18 percent. Levels of seven key nutrients were analyzed in the study, and the only one to increase in potatoes over the fifty-year period was niacin.[8]

Is it any wonder that we veterinarians now routinely examine young dogs with terminal cancer and other chronic, degenerative diseases? I'm convinced that man created degenerative disease.

Years ago, if a dog ate a certain amount of liver and adrenals each week, he would get the full quota of vitamins and minerals intended to be derived from these foods to maintain his health. If you took that same dog today, however, and fed him the same amount of liver and adrenals, the dog's nutrition would be deficient.

Why? There are two main reasons.

First, the animals that the organs were harvested from to be used in the dog's food were themselves nutritionally deficient. You would have to feed the dog far more liver and adrenals for him to get the full quota of vitamins and minerals required for good health.

Second, the dog himself can no longer process his food at peak efficiency. Due to the degradation of the environment caused by humans, the gene pools of dogs and other animals—including we humans—have become debilitated. The digestive systems don't work as well, and what nutrients are there aren't being fully taken up and utilized by cells.

How can we make up for that deficiency? By giving our animals foods in concentrated form—also known as *nutraceuticals*.

As an integrative veterinarian, I treat dogs, cats, and other animals with whatever substance or treatment my many years of experience tells me will have the greatest chance of maintaining or restoring good health. Remember, my job as a veterinarian is not to "cure" our animal companions, it's to guide them toward health, then get out of the way and allow Mother Nature to do what she does best.

ASK DR. MARTY

Q: Are most supplements such as vitamins and minerals all basically the same, or are there quality differences that have the potential to make a difference in the health and well-being of my animal companion?

A: Many years ago, in my early quest to learn about the health benefits of nutrition, I came upon a controlled study that was performed on lab rats. I recently scoured the internet to find a copy of this study to include as a citation, but was unsuccessful. Here's what I recall:

All of the rats were made deficient in iron and then divided into three groups.

The diet of the first group remained completely devoid of iron, and they all died.

The diet of the second group was supplemented with an inorganic form of iron—I believe ferrous oxide or ferrous sulfate. A low percentage of the animals—less than 30 percent—recovered.

With the third and final group, the same inorganic iron fed to the second group of lab animals was first placed in the soil in which carrots were grown. Then the carrots were ground up and fed to this third group. Surprisingly, more than 90 percent recovered.

When I studied under Dr. Bernard Jensen, one of the all-time great modern healers, he shared a similar story with me from when he worked at a chicken farm in Oakland, California. No matter how much they supplemented the feed with calcium, the chickens were not vibrant, and their eggs cracked easily during the delivery process—leading to much product waste. After studying the success of chicken farmers in Petaluma, California—then considered the "egg capital of the world"—he found that the feed they used was being supplemented with green kale, which has a naturally very high calcium content. When Dr. Jensen added kale to his own chicken feed, egg breakage diminished tremendously, and the egg yolks became much richer and darker in color.[9]

This was a major wake-up call for me in the science of supplementation. And a game changer for maintaining my own health. I learned that there was a lot more to the effective use of nutraceuticals than just ingesting the scientific numerical amount of an essential nutrient listed on a label. These two studies demonstrated the beneficial difference between unchelated and chelated nutrients. The word *chelate* means "claw," and in the case of the inorganic chemical iron placed in the soil, the uptake into the carrots chelated this iron into the plant's protein matrix, making it so much more organically bioavailable.

So, yes, there is a big difference between synthetic, man-made supplements that I would consider to be chemicals, and nutraceuticals that are derived from food sources that are organically raised. I am also not a great fan of the word *natural*. As I always say, "Lead is natural. Would you eat it?"

BIOLOGICAL VERSUS SYNTHETIC NUTRACEUTICALS

I'm often asked if it's okay for pet parents to feed their loved ones any type of synthetic nutraceutical. My answer is no—that you should always seek out naturally harvested sources of nutrition wherever possible, and that includes in the use of nutraceuticals.

During my visit to Switzerland, I discovered a unique family of food-grade nutraceuticals made by a Zurich-based company called Bio-Strath. The nutraceuticals are made from Strath's proprietary formula of specially processed herbal yeast (*Saccharomyces cerevisiae*), and other plant-based ingredients including angelica root, lemon-balm leaf, chamomile flower, cinnamon bark, caraway seed, elder flower, fennel seed, horseradish root, hyssop leaf, lavender flower, parsley aerial parts, peppermint leaf, sage leaf, and thyme aerial parts. These plant-based ingredients are added at a specific time in the yeast's fermentation to maximize their biological activity. This stuff is so good that, even now, I take it almost every day.

Bio-Strath also produces a line of nutraceuticals specifically for animals called Anima-Strath, which, according to the company, increase immune defenses, increase vitality, promote metabolism, provide a healthy, glossy coat or plumage, maintain health and well-being, and more.

When I was in Zurich, I contacted Bio-Strath, and they were happy to give me a tour of their manufacturing operation, including where they ferment the yeast they use in their different products. It was all quite impressive.

There's something special about Switzerland, and I think it has a lot to do with their not having degraded their cropland to the same degree that we have in the United States. During the three days I was there, I regularly visited a small stand on the street that sold the freshest, most vital produce you've ever seen in your life. One day I bought what I thought was a basket of plums. Paying for the fruit, I asked, "What kind of plums are these?" In broken English, the woman replied, "No, those aren't plums, they're grapes." I couldn't believe it—they were huge, and beautiful. And these weren't artificial, GMO-enhanced fruit. The grapes were huge because they were so healthy.

It was the same thing with some lettuce I bought at the stand. It was like no other lettuce I had ever seen back home. The first day, I peeled off a couple of one-and-a-half-foot-long, dark green leaves and ate them. They weren't the pale, light green and yellow lettuce leaves that you'll find in your neighborhood supermarket. The chlorophyll was all there. The second day, I tore away the rest of the outer leaves—hungrily eating them. Long green shoots had pushed out, then dived back into the center of the plant. It was amazing, and it tasted vital, healthy, alive. By the third day, I got to the core, and it looked familiar—like a big ball. I went back to the stand to ask the woman, "What kind of lettuce is this? I've never seen anything like it."

"Iceberg."

All I can say is that what we call iceberg lettuce in the United States is a pale imitation of the real thing—with all the nutrition and flavor bred out of it to make it easy for farmers to harvest, transport, and store.

The entire time I was in Switzerland, I was continuously amazed at just how healthy the Swiss people looked. Eighty percent of the people I saw—especially the teenagers and the twenty-year-olds—could have been cover models. They were healthy, fit, and robust with perfect posture and physiques. They glowed from within and were always smiling. They were the human versions of the grapes and the iceberg lettuce I had bought from that little stand down the street from my hotel.

Contrast that to the day I flew back home to New York. When I arrived at the airport, I discovered that the flight was delayed for about two and a half hours. So, while I waited for my flight to board, I just sat and people-watched. As the group of people flying back to the United States gathered and milled about in the gate area, I immediately noticed a distinct contrast with the Swiss people I had encountered on the street while I was in Zurich. Instead of the picture of health and happiness that the Swiss airport employees were displaying right in front of me, the Americans in line were modeling something quite different. Many were unhealthy looking, overweight, bald, screaming, yelling, unhappy. I thought to myself, "I don't want to go back."

I'm convinced that the Swiss looked so vital and alive because of their food chain. I saw firsthand just how great the native food is and has been for millennia in Switzerland, and just how poor the food is that most of us eat here in the United States. Because of our poor food chain, we sure need nutraceuticals to compensate. And so do our animal companions—the dogs and cats that have become much-loved and cherished members of our families.

Years ago, I was asked to write articles for a health magazine that circulated in New York City. Each issue had an overall theme, and my topic on pet health care needed to stay within that theme. One time when I received an invitation to contribute an article, the subject matter for the issue was "the environment." Hmmm. I wondered, "Besides the age-old dangers of environmental toxins, what could I come up with?" With the vision I'd brought back from Switzerland—a vision that stuck so deeply within me—I came up with something I call the *anatomy of destruction*.

THE ANATOMY OF DESTRUCTION

Let's take ourselves to the beginning of man's stay here on earth, and let's make the assumption that things were running (as they most likely were) just fine. There wasn't the degree of disease as we know it today—cancer, heart disease, and other common maladies. Also, no industrial pollution, insecticides, germicides, pesticides, and the rest of the "cides"—the killers—that pervade our modern environment.

Life used to be much simpler—and in many ways better. People hunted and they gathered, and they learned to farm. These early people had a routine: sow the seeds that their plants produced every year, tend their gardens and their animals, eat the food that they produced, and use the raw materials that nature provided. People lived their lives in harmony with the world around them. They were acutely aware of the forces of nature, and they worked *with* instead of *against* them.

But it's deep within human nature to constantly improve and become more affluent, typically for reasons of self-betterment. So, people began to harness the forces of nature for their own benefit—not foreseeing the end results of their actions because of their limited consciousness. Even when they could foresee the end results, they would often break their mutually agreed-upon rules of ethics to rationalize their actions, with society invariably taking a nosedive.

Now, let's see how this theory applies to illness.

A healthy being, be it human or animal, lives in an environment filled with billions of bacteria, viruses, insects, and much more, but no disease exists. It's a place of health and harmony. Then, this being doesn't take care of itself, and the bacteria that normally coexisted in her throat with no consequence start to multiply, and she gets a "sore throat." Or, through the feeding of an improper diet of processed, preserved, and imbalanced foods, fleas start to "attack" a weakened dog or cat.

Now, here is where the destructive process, instead of being remedied, accelerates rapidly.

With only rare exceptions, there really is nothing new on the earth or, for that matter, in the universe. Therefore, no matter how new a substance or product might appear to be, it is always composed of that which is already here. So, scientists take naturally occurring elements and compounds of the earth (remember the periodic table of elements from high school?) and put them together in aberrated or twisted formulas that render them highly toxic to life and to the earth itself.

In a balanced and natural world, your dog or cat would have fleas but not be affected by them—they would coexist. Unfortunately, that's not the case for much of the world today, and fleas can be a real problem. But, instead of educating you on correct diet and care to help your pet return to a proper coexistence with fleas, scientists instead develop highly toxic chemicals from already existing, relatively inert substances. These powerful chemicals destroy the fleas, typically using your animal companion as the delivery system.

Awareness ends right there. You spray your dog or cat, you give it a pill or apply a tube of liquid, or you set off a couple of flea bombs in your house. For a short time, your flea problem is resolved, but the fleas inevitably return, and the flea problem for your animal companion is usually worse. It's a temporary fix at best.

And what happens to those chemicals? They don't just go away or disappear. They end up back in the environment with their full toxic potential intact.

What about the treatment of cancer with chemotherapy? You take a body with an already-weakened immune system that can't properly maintain itself, and you bombard it with some of the most powerful chemicals in medicine. You do this in hopes of destroying cancerous cells while preserving the healthy cells. However, the typical sequel in patients who survive this process is the return of the cancer months or years later. Treatment commences once again, and patients are often sucked into even harsher regimens of therapy, further weakening their already-depleted bodies.

And where do these powerful chemicals go after they are consumed by the body? They don't stop there! They get urinated, defecated, salivated, or sweated out into the environment, or they get stored in the body's cells only to be released upon burial after death or directly into the atmosphere upon cremation.

We follow the irrational logic of taking from the earth, converting natural substances into toxins, then constantly recycling them into the environment: physical life, the earth on which we exist, and the atmosphere that surrounds us. This, in my opinion, is the real cause of cancer. The lumps or malignancies that occur in our bodies are just a side effect of this misguided mechanism.

And what about radiation? For diagnosis and therapy,

medical science tends to use those wavelengths from many parts of the electromagnetic spectrum that specifically exclude the part in which life functions and thrives: visible light. Expensive equipment has been created to produce or concentrate gamma rays, X-rays, radiation, magnetic resonance, and more, then focus them on diseased bodies—subjecting them to concentrated vibrational frequencies to which they are not accustomed. More toxicity, but now of a higher form and typically more potent.

Do these rays stop there? I wonder. Now we are creating even more atmospheric pollution, and of a much higher and more dangerous form. Remember Newton's third law of motion: for every action, there is an equal and opposite reaction. When you take the action of concentrating radiation and shooting it out into our environment, what is the inevitable equal and opposite reaction?

So, what's the answer to this ever-tighter spiral of destruction that we have created?

Simple! Take from the earth those substances that are native and administer them to those who have, by their disease process, gone out of balance with their environment. Create and support a science geared to study and develop methods of practice knowing which products or procedures, and in what combinations, will enhance this healing process in the most efficient and expeditious way. Fit this practice in with current, conventional practice as an adjunct and watch it take over as society improves.

This is the beating heart of integrative veterinary medicine, and it's what I have dedicated my life to achieving.

A WORD ABOUT DR. GOOGLE

In the sections that follow, I'm going to explore some of what I think are the most important and most effective nutraceuticals available for our animal companions. So many nutraceuticals are available today—with more coming out all the time—that it's not humanly possible to keep up with all of them. In addition to the ones that follow, I suggest you explore the many others via the internet—probably the number one resource for medical advice on the planet.

One caveat, however: before you try out some new nutraceutical on your animal companion based on Dr. Google's advice, be sure to work closely with an integrative veterinarian—someone you trust and who takes the time to get to know the dogs or cats in your life. If you're not sure where to find an experienced integrative veterinarian in your area, you can do a search on the website of the American Holistic Veterinary Medical Association (AHVMA): www.ahvma.org.

Keep in mind that there isn't just one treatment or approach or regimen—no silver bullet—to make or keep a patient healthy. There can be different paths to the same goal—all equally valid, all equally effective—including changing the diet, taking nutraceuticals, exercise, fasting, and much more. I'm reminded of when I trained my first veterinarian. After eight or nine months, she took a two-week vacation, and in her absence I covered the cases she was working on. Right before I was going to examine one of her patients, I reviewed the dog's records. The nutraceuticals my veterinarian trainee had prescribed were not the ones I would have chosen based on what I had taught her. I thought to myself, "Oh, God—I need to spend more time teaching this young veterinarian how to do things the right way!"

So, I knocked on the door of the exam room and stepped inside, where I was greeted with a happy-looking dog and her pet parent. "So, how is she doing?" I asked.

"Oh my God—she's doing great!" was the pet parent's immediate reply. "She's never been this healthy!"

At that moment, I realized that there's more than one way—*my* way—to get healthy. Different veterinarians will take different approaches, based on their unique combinations of knowledge, experience, and practice, along with the unique characteristics and medical history of the patient in front of them. Your job as a loving and conscientious pet parent is to find the best veterinarian for your animal companions you can.

While the internet is a great place to get general medical advice and information on different nutraceuticals and when and how they are used, it can never replace a good veterinarian who personally knows his or her patients. There's just no comparison. That flood of information you'll encounter on the internet—some based on real research, and some untested and unproven—can make it a challenge to make good decisions on behalf of your animal companions.

MEDICINAL MUSHROOMS

Mushrooms are interesting organisms. You've heard of the two main kingdoms on our planet—the animal kingdom and the plant kingdom. Some believe that mushrooms belong to a third kingdom separate from the animal and the plant kingdoms. Here's an excerpt from a book on the cancer-fighting properties of maitake mushrooms:

> Mushrooms and other fungi have been called "the third kingdom." Being neither plant nor animal, they are a world unto themselves. Their genetic make-up is actually closer to that of humans and animals than to plants. (We share approximately 30 percent of our DNA with mushrooms.)[10]

So much has been written on the positive effects of medicinal mushrooms, and most of that writing is by people who are currently doing research into their beneficial effects. As I was researching for this book the scientific studies on medicinal mushrooms, one of the first references I found was an article published in *Oncotarget*—a peer-reviewed medical journal that focuses on oncology (the study of cancer). Here's an excerpt from the abstract of the article:

> Medicinal mushrooms have been used throughout the history of mankind for treatment of various diseases including cancer. Nowadays they have been intensively studied in order to reveal the chemical nature and mechanisms of action of their biomedical capacity. Targeted treatment of cancer, nonharmful for healthy tissues, has become a desired goal in recent decades and compounds of fungal origin provide a vast reservoir of potential innovational drugs.[11]

Then there's this study, which comes to us from the University of Pennsylvania School of Veterinary Medicine. It deals with one of the most tragic and least responsive cancers dogs can possibly get: hemangiosarcoma—a cancer that has reached almost epidemic status. According to a University of Pennsylvania news release on the research findings:

> Dogs with hemangiosarcoma that were treated with a compound derived from the *Coriolus versicolor* mushroom had the longest survival times ever reported for dogs with the disease. These promising findings offer hope that the compound may one day offer cancer patients—human and canine alike—a viable alternative or complementary treatment to traditional chemotherapies.[12]

What blows me away is that, after I have been fighting for the acceptance and use of these sorts of nutraceuticals for so many years, the highest echelon of conventional medicine is now talking my language.

The mushroom in the study, *Coriolus versicolor*, a staple in Chinese medicine for thousands of years, is also known as the turkey tail mushroom. According to Dorothy Cimino Brown, one of the researchers who published the study, "We were shocked. Prior to this, the longest-reported median survival time of dogs with hemangiosarcoma of the spleen that underwent no further treatment was eighty-six days. We had dogs that lived beyond a year with nothing other than this mushroom as treatment."[13] They were so shocked that they asked the Penn veterinary pathologists to recheck the results, which were indeed confirmed correct.

Of the many medicinal mushrooms, each has specific beneficial effects. These can easily be researched. In general, the potential benefits related to the entire category of medicinal mushrooms are:

- Antioxidant (fight free radicals—compounds that cause damage to cells and DNA)
- Longevity
- Immunity
- Anti-inflammatory
- Antibacterial
- Antiviral
- Antistress
- Anti-fatigue
- Energy
- Heart health
- Liver protection
- Digestive issue
- Skin conditions
- Sleep and mood issues
- Hormonal balance support
- Adrenal support
- Anticancer

When eaten as food, these mushrooms are a source of essential vitamins, pro-vitamins, minerals, and trace minerals. They contain an important complex polysaccharide molecule called beta-glucan, which scientific evidence says supports antitumor activity and the immune system. Of the numerous medicinal mushrooms, here are the ones that I particularly like:

- Chaga—the King of the Mushrooms
- Coriolus (turkey tail)
- Reishi
- Shiitake
- Lion's mane
- Cordyceps
- Maitake

For fifteen years, I have used in clinical practice a liquid maitake supplement for my patients called PETfraction—produced by Mushroom Wisdom, Inc. About eight years ago, the company flew representatives to visit me at Smith Ridge, and they showed me scientific documentation of tumor regression solely from use of this supplement. Then, a few years back, Mushroom Wisdom's mother company flew me to Japan to lecture to 350 veterinarians at four different veterinary conferences in three different cities.

I was honored when I was told afterward that, in this kind of conference, usually 30 percent of the audience leaves the room to seek out other presentations of more interest, but almost nobody left mine. Also, questions are rarely asked by the attendees after any talk at these conferences, but the audience stayed and asked me quite a few after each of my presentations. And I did everything through an interpreter.

I was joined by a veterinary oncologist from the veterinary

school in Tokyo, who presented documentation demonstrating increased lymphocyte numbers against cancer in those taking this mushroom-fraction supplement. I was even more impressed.

HERBS AND PLANTS

Herbs are an integral part of our natural world, and they have been used by humans for many thousands of years. Many herbs are highly medicinal—the closest thing to a drug without the bad side effects—and they can have strong anti-inflammatory, antiallergy, and immune-supportive effects in our animal companions. Some herbs can actually help break down cancer.

We all know that the gel in the aloe vera plant can be used to treat burns, including sunburns. It also has tremendous nutritional effects for the body. It's high in amino acids, and it can ease digestion while speeding up intestinal detoxification. It's anti-inflammatory, especially when used topically for burns, allergies, and rashes. I have always recommended that every household should have at least one live aloe vera plant—not only to treat the dogs and cats in our lives, but also for their human parents. And last but not least, aloe vera has shown potential as an anticancer treatment. According to the Susan G. Komen website, "There is preliminary evidence that aloe consumption may reduce the risk of lung cancer or tumor growth. Further research is needed in this area."[14]

The huge field of herbs offers a vast array of choices. In

general, the two main categories are Western herbs and those of the Far East—specifically Chinese. Although each specific herb within each category has its own medicinal properties, I have always leaned toward using combination formulas.

With so many possible herbs and combinations of herbs, my number one bit of advice is to work with a practitioner who is well versed in their usage, especially when using the Chinese formulas loaded with at least a dozen herbs—few of which any of us can even pronounce.

And one last thought when it comes to this classification of supplementation. I feel that society as a whole took a huge downward turn when we scientifically isolated the active ingredients in plant medicinals—such as we did with digitalis for heart conditions, which was originally extracted from the dried leaves of foxglove plants—and started manufacturing them in pharmaceutical factories, often with more toxic effects (including, in the case of digitalis, the condition called digitalis toxicity).

ESSENTIAL FATTY ACIDS

These are near the top of the list of importance for nutritional supplementation for pets as they are vital for the proper functioning and health of the heart, liver, kidneys, eyes, skin and coat, digestive system, and joints. They also help regulate inflammatory pathways in the body and protect against allergies and even cancer.

The two main types of essential fatty acids (EFAs) are omega-3 and omega-6. In general, omega-3 EFAs are considered anti-inflammatory, while the omega-6 EFAs are considered pro-inflammatory—that is, they promote inflammation instead of hindering it. Both of these fatty acids are called essential because you and your animal companions cannot produce them in your bodies—they must be ingested. We need the proper balance of omega-3 and omega-6 fatty acids, however. Omega-3s are anti-inflammatory, anti-allergy, and provide immune support. When the concentration of omega-6 fatty acids is too high, this can actually create inflammation.

What's usually considered optimal, especially for our canine companions, is a ratio of 4:1 or 5:1 omega-6 to omega-3. Surprisingly, many commercial pet foods have a ratio of around 20:1, and with the many corn-based foods, it can go as high as 50:1. I am convinced this is one of the main reasons I have over my career witnessed such a huge escalation of inflammatory diseases.

But this assumes that EFAs make it into pet food at all. Not only are EFAs easily destroyed by the heating processes used throughout the pet food industry, but they are highly unstable and easily break down in the presence of oxygen—a process called oxidation. Not only does this render them fairly useless, but they can turn rancid, rendering them toxic to health.

The two best sources of these omega-3 and omega-6 fatty acids are fish and krill—a tiny crustacean that looks like a miniature, two-inch-long lobster without claws. In addition, coconut oil is lately getting positive reviews, especially for dogs. But there is also controversy—recent research indicates that feeding coconut oil to dogs may cause problems.[15]

So many products containing essential fatty acids are available today that I'm not going to recommend any particular brands. Just make sure the ones you choose are from a reputable company that guarantees their freshness and stability. For proper dosing, it would also help if you get one specifically formulated for pets, as these should have a correct dose-per-weight chart right on the label.

One caveat: As beneficial as I have seen both fish and krill oil to be in clinical practice over many years with my patients, a number of negatives have been reported. A particularly important one is that many fish oil sources turn rancid by oxidation by the time the product reaches your pet's mouth.[16] Also, these oils are a potential source of toxins and heavy-metal poisons.[17]

Added to this are ecological concerns that I will not touch upon.

While the established benefits of the omega-3 components of these oils are compelling, the controversy around them has led me to strongly look at other, safer sources such as phytoplankton, algae, and hemp oil.

The dosing for these fatty acids in a cancer or allergy patient is a lot higher than just maintenance. Dosing is done according to the label and according to the condition—working with your veterinarian. We usually start with low, acclimating doses and work our way up from there. In a patient with cancer or a severe allergy, we go up to what's called bowel tolerance—you slowly increase the dose of the oil you give, day by day, until the patient's stool gets a little loose. Then you back down a little. The more you give, the better. But you'll need to consult with your veterinarian to get the dosage right—he or she knows your dog or cat, I don't.

DIGESTIVE ENZYMES

Another medical therapy that is gaining traction in the treatment of dogs and cats is digestive enzymes. They are very, very important. I consider them a food because without them food is not properly utilized by the body—it's not broken down. Also, biologically raw food tends to have a high content of these enzymes within the food itself, which gets released and aids in digestion. Cooking food instantly diminishes enzyme content. Our dog or cat can eat the finest food in the world, but if the digestive enzymes created by the pancreas, stomach, and the lining of the intestines are not properly breaking down the food, it's not going to be effectively absorbed and utilized.

More specifically, *proteolytic* enzymes—including peptidases, proteases, or proteinases—break down protein in the digestive tract. The orthodontist and dentist Dr. William Donald Kelley used high levels of digestive enzymes, especially proteolytic enzymes, to break down cancer cells in humans.

In my own practice, we started to use these enzymes decades ago with dogs and cats, and we saw a positive effect in shrinking or breaking down tumors.

ARTEMISININ

Artemisinin is a natural remedy that has been used in China for thousands of years. The compound is derived from *Artemisia annua*, the sweet wormwood plant, and it has been traditionally prescribed as a treatment for malaria and other parasitic infections. According to the World Health Organization website, "Artemisinin and its derivatives are powerful medicines known for their ability to swiftly reduce the number of *Plasmodium* parasites [the vector for malaria] in the blood of patients with malaria."[18] In 2015, scientist Tu Youyou was awarded the Nobel Prize for her discovery of artemisinin and her use of it to treat malaria—saving millions of lives. Now, that's *real* medicine.

My understanding is that artemisinin interacts with iron, causing a release of free-radical compounds that are cytotoxic, or deadly to cells. The malaria organism likes iron, and where it is taken up by the organism (called ferro-receptor sites), these free radicals get released and kill the organism.

Guess what else likes iron? Yup, cancer.

Perhaps it's no surprise then that it's been scientifically proven that artemisinin is an anticancer therapeutic. Chemotherapy and radiation typically have the same cancer-killing mechanism, but obviously this compound—derived from natural plant sources—would prove to be a lot less toxic and free of adverse reactions compared to these conventional modalities.

I have been using artemisinin as one of the main anticancer preparations in my arsenal. And there's a bonus: artemisinin is also pretty effective in helping treat tick-borne diseases such as Lyme disease. I can vouch for that from personal and family experience.

GLANDULARS

For decades, we have used glandular supplements to treat dog and cat disease. These substances are taken from a variety of mammalian organs and tissues, for example, from the pancreas, thyroid, adrenals, thymus, and many others. Glandulars have been effective in our practice, and it makes sense—especially when you consider that in nature dogs and cats ate all the organs when they killed their prey for food. We'll use concentrated glandulars to help reestablish health and metabolic function.

Although their main mechanism of action would be considered as "like helps like," the more accepted one is that when an organ becomes diseased, the body makes antibodies against it. The glandular acts as a decoy for the immune system to attack—leaving the native organ be so it can heal.

THE CBD CRAZE

Yes, craze. I get at least three spam emails a day offering for sale all sorts of miraculous CBD-related products for me and my pets. This is a subject rather near and dear to my heart. When I was in college—especially a place such as Cornell in the sixties and early seventies—it was tough *not* to partake of one form of cannabis or another! Although all that has been gone from my life for at least the past thirty years, I'm glad I had the experience. So, it's probably no surprise that I'm thrilled about all the current research around CBD—a naturally occurring, plant-based substance—and its documented beneficial effects for the animal kingdom.

One of the closest, long-term colleagues I have in this holistic veterinary community is my buddy Dr. Rob Silver. He's from Boulder, Colorado—the place I once thought I was going to move to and set up shop. Like me, Rob is one of the "founding elders" in the American Holistic Veterinary Medical Association. Even better, when I was the lead singer in the AHVMA band—we performed at the big annual conference each year—Rob was my lead acoustic guitarist.

But even more important, Rob was responsible for starting up one of the first (and I would maintain *best*) nutraceutical companies focused on pets. Rob's company, Rx Vitamins for Pets, developed groundbreaking products that gained widespread acceptance in our profession—not an easy thing to do. More recently, he has turned his attention solely to the research and development of, and worldwide education for, CBD products for dogs and cats, with a particular focus on the medical science substantiating CBD's value.

When I lectured with Dr. Ian Billinghurst in Canada, Rob completed the triad of keynote speakers, and I was blown away by his talks. Who better to invite to write a piece on this topic?

PET CBD: AN EXCITING EMERGING THERAPY FOR PETS

BY ROBERT J. SILVER, DVM, MS

I graduated from Colorado State University's Veterinary College in 1982, and I've been in small animal practice in Boulder since 1993. I practiced in Colorado during the time medical marijuana and adult recreational-use marijuana were legalized in the state, and from that experience, as a holistic veterinarian and as a veterinary medical herbalist, I learned how effective cannabis can be to treat medical problems in our pets, which even advanced holistic therapies such as Marty and I used daily in our practices could not touch.

I learned from these early experiences with medical marijuana that dogs are very, very sensitive to the unbalancing and intoxicating effects of tetrahydrocannabinol (THC)—the molecule in the cannabis plant that is still not kosher for veterinarians to recommend because, at the federal level, it is still illegal. Some dogs who get too much THC will have problems with it and often find themselves at the animal ER sleeping it off, although there are a few reports of dogs dying from "overdoses" of THC. Those reports also indicate that in addition to the overdose of THC, these dogs also ingested a lot of chocolate, which is quite toxic to dogs.

In 2014, the US government passed a law (the Farm Bill) allowing the legal cultivation and commercialization of hemp, which is cannabis that is not intoxicating since it contains such a small amount of THC, and in some cases nearly no THC. Hemp is, however, high in CBD. This is an exciting development because CBD has revolutionized efforts to address some difficult problems in pets and has shown itself to be both safe and effective at low or "microdoses" with no intoxicating effects.

In 2018, the US government passed an updated farm bill that further legalized the use of CBD from hemp. Since then, we have seen in the marketplace a large number of start-ups offering what they call "pet CBD oil," with many claims for their products to cure many different diseases.

Several veterinary studies have been conducted, and from those we have seen that CBD can be helpful with the loss of mobility in dogs with osteoarthritis. Another study showed that CBD can help with epilepsy, although not as much as we have been hoping for at the doses they used in the study.

Nonetheless, pet owners have been reporting on social media and other media outlets that their dogs have been responding well to pet CBD oil for a variety of issues, including anxiety, pain, indigestion, epilepsy, arthritis, and even some types of cancer.

Here are some things to know if you are thinking about trying CBD oil for your pet:

- Not all products are what they say they are. Some companies that have jumped on the CBD oil bandwagon to make a buck are using oil that may not have CBD in it at all or may contain toxins from solvents used in the extraction of the CBD oil or from other sources.

- Consumers need to ask companies for a certificate of analysis (CoA) from a third-party laboratory that is certified by the state to have high standards of quality control. This document will tell you not just how much CBD is in the oil but will also reassure you that the THC in the product is low enough to not get your pet high. This document will also inform you if any contaminants, such as heavy metals, pesticides, yeast, mold, or solvent residues, were found in the oil. If so, I suggest you find a different company with a better-quality oil.
- If the company tells you they won't show you the CoA, that is a clear indication to look elsewhere for your CBD oil.
- Guidelines for dosing your dog or cat are simple:
  - For the anxious pet, you should give about 0.1 mg for each pound of body weight, twice daily. In some cases, if that doesn't work after seven to ten days, you may need to double that dose to get a better effect.
  - For the pet with mobility issues, a higher dose of 0.25 mg per pound of body weight to 0.5 mg per pound, twice daily, is likely to help.
  - Some types of cancer and epilepsy will respond to CBD oil at the higher dosing ranges, but not all will respond as much as we might like. So, it's always worth a try to see if this emerging therapy can help your pet, versus using drugs that may have adverse side effects.
  - It's hard to predict how an individual pet will respond to CBD oil. The best way is to try it for seven

to fourteen days at a lower dose, and if after two weeks you aren't getting the results you want, then double or quadruple the dose. We know that in at least one study doses up to 5 mg per pound for six weeks have been proven safe.

- You can give the oil by simply squirting it into the mouth, where it will be absorbed through the mucous membranes. Not all pets will allow that, so you can also put the dose on a small amount of "bribe food" in between meals, and that will be absorbed about as well.

To conclude, CBD oil is being used successfully by pet parents to help their pets with a variety of problems. It has shown itself to be relatively safe when given at the accepted lower dosages suggested here. CBD oil may not treat every problem out there, but it has been shown to help with many.

DIGESTIVE HEALTH

As I wrote earlier, although we may accept the old saying "We are what we eat," much more significant is "We are what we *metabolize*." What happens to the food in the GI tract is vital to health, and much focus now is on what's called the *microbiome*. I recently attended a talk on this topic at my alma mater, the Cornell College of Veterinary Medicine, given by my dear colleague Dr. Rick Palmquist. Here's the introduction to his talk, which I reproduce with his permission:

We are now discovering and consciously interacting with a strange new world, the world of the microbiome, a virtual organ that acts locally and globally and holds tremendous promise in managing and preventing some of the most challenging categories of disease we face in our clinics.

Historically, we defined the microbiome as the populations of specific microorganisms in a particular environment. We depend upon a vast army of microorganisms to stay alive; a microbiome that breaks down food to release energy and produces vitamins, antioxidants, short chain fatty acids, essential amino acids, and a wide variety of useful substances. Using this definition, we developed only limited understanding of a few components of the microbiome. To cover this definition, we now use the term microbiota. Species are categorized by their relationship to the host: *probionts* are synergistic; *commensals* live with the host in harmony; and *pathobionts* are potentially harmful and associated with disease.

A healthy dog's microbiome is vastly different from an ill dog's, and the microbiome is in constant fluctuation, a factor that means that we never see the same "patient" twice. Every case is changing from one visit to the next. Astute clinicians can observe these changes in odor, tartar, stool character, skin and ear changes, and several other issues. There is now evidence that Chinese tongue diagnosis links to such changes in the microbiome and resultant physiology of the patient.

We now view the microbiome in a more cohesive and useful way as "the combined genetic material of the microorganisms of a particular environment"; e.g., "understanding the microbiome is as important as understanding the human genome." Fundamentally, while we are discussing the total population of microorganisms (bacteria, protozoa, fungi, and viruses) present in a single organic identity, this term encompasses the total genomic aspects of this community. It is not just the summary of the total number of individual organisms, but their activity from a genomic aspect. This genomic understanding gives us an inkling of the massive scope of this field and how it interrelates to homeostasis, pathogenesis, and potential recovery. As microorganisms flow from soil to plants and animals, this subject connects life in a dynamic and responsive way. It is important to note that recent research is uncovering microbial inhabitants in organs beside the gut including the eye, womb, placenta, lung, and brain.

So how do we support proper gut health? Probiotics have gained wide popularity even in the human health field in recent years, and I am a big fan. How can you tell if your dog has good gut health? Eating grass is my Canine Distress Call #1.

You may have been told that dogs swallow grass when they ate something bad, to make themselves throw up. In my experience, "dogs eat grass because they ate something bad" is a myth. Studies show less than 25 percent of dogs throw up at all when they eat grass.

So why do pets eat grass?

I believe this distress call is saying one major thing: "I have an imbalance in my gut." Now, your dog doesn't know what an "intestinal imbalance" is, but your dog's body does know when something is wrong. Eating grass is one way dogs try to remedy this!

All living creatures have bacteria inside their bodies, especially in their intestines. According to the US National Institutes of Health, the average human has about five pounds of bacteria in his or her gut at any time. And there's basically two kinds of bacteria: good and bad.

The good bacteria are important to our health, as they impact how we break down food and even affect our mood, our immune system, and our overall health.

The bad bacteria, on the other hand, can make us hungrier than we should be and contribute to weight gain, mood swings, allergies, and even sickness.

So, in every mammal, the goal is to have a balance of mostly good bacteria in the gut. This is true for humans—and even more so for dogs. Why is gut health so important for dogs? Because dogs can't control what they eat. If your body is craving good bacteria, it might send messages to your brain to eat more yogurt, cheese, kimchi, or sauerkraut. These might seem like random foods, but they're all packed with good bacteria, and when you eat them, you'll often feel better!

But your dog?

Unfortunately, most dogs eat the same food every day. They can't go "shopping" for something different when they have an urge—they can't even tell you what the urge is!

But they *will* experience the symptoms of a gut imbalance, such as:

- Poor digestion
- Flatulence
- Poor mood and fatigue
- Anxiousness
- And even weight gain

As you can imagine, dogs don't like these signs. And this is why dogs eat grass. Because in the wild, grass is usually full of good bacteria. So this is how your dog "shops" for gut-friendly food! A number of studies have shown that children who play in grass and dirt more as kids go on to have healthier GI tracts, develop fewer allergies, and even are less likely to experience IBS and autoimmune diseases.

You may also notice dogs eat more grass in the beginning of spring. This is sort of like a dog's version of "spring cleaning." After a long winter, when many dogs sleep a lot and their metabolism slows down—they need to "clean out" their GI tract.

So, what can you do to help your dog rebalance her gut?

Eating more grass is not the answer. Yes, in the wild, grass can contain helpful bacteria. But in suburbs and cities, where grass and dirt are exposed to pesticides, weed killers, and other toxins? Grass can make a gut imbalance worse.

If your dog is tolerant of fermented forms of dairy, such as yogurt, I recommend a spoonful of natural Greek yogurt as a way to get probiotics into its system. You can also use natural probiotic-rich foods such as sauerkraut, although many dogs won't eat this. That's why I feel the best solution is a purified source of good bacteria—also known as probiotics. You may have heard about probiotics before. These good bacteria usually come in pill, capsule, or powder form, and when ingested, they go to work in your dog's digestive system. Here, they crowd out the bad bacteria, rebalancing the proper flora.

In humans as well as dogs, probiotics have been shown to provide *all* of the following:

- Healthier digestion
- Less gas
- Better immune system
- Better-smelling bowel movements
- More energy
- Even better mood

There's one more thing you should know. While probiotics are good bacteria, there's something called *prebiotics*, which are what good bacteria like to eat. To keep your dog's "good bacteria" strong, you should give them the stuff that helps them multiply and destroy bad bacteria.

This is why I love prebiotics. They're indigestible, so they're guaranteed to go straight to your dog's colon, where the good bacteria are. And they only get eaten by the good bacteria, not the bad! Using prebiotics is like sending an "airmail" package of supplies to your good bacteria behind enemy lines, giving them the tools they need to fight on your dog's behalf!

So, what are the best sources of prebiotics for dogs? In nature, dogs can find them in certain wild plants and other sources. But as we've discussed, the modern world just doesn't have healthy sources of these plants in abundance— and when you do find them, they've probably been doused with tons of pesticides, chemicals, or other toxins that make them more harmful than good. This is why I like good prebiotic supplementation.

I'm a big fan of medicinal mushrooms. An extract made from champignon mushrooms goes by the name of Champex. Mushrooms are well-known immune boosters and can help reduce oxidative stress on the body. They're also great for boosting brain health. But what really got me excited was a landmark study at Penn State that showed these beneficial effects of mushrooms may be from one specific thing they do: the researchers found mushrooms improve the balance of bacteria in the gut.

In one experiment, researchers found that elderly people at a Japanese health care facility given champignon-mushroom extract

> showed a significant improvement in stool odor and stool color, and an improvement in quality of life (satisfaction) was expressed. More specifically, stool odor, which is one of the bowel movement problems in elderly people, was alleviated by champignon extract, suggesting an improvement in quality of life associated with bowel movement.[19]

After researchers ran multiple lab tests on Champex for its safety in canines, I began giving it to dogs suffering from bad odors, smelly poop, flatulence, loose stool, excessive tartar buildup, bad breath, dental issues, itching, or red eyes and ears. In short, any dogs that had the telltale "distress calls" of gut imbalances.

When dogs started taking this formula, they didn't just do well. They thrived—some of them for the first time in years. Even young dogs got the gut health they needed—achieving the true healthy spirit they always had inside them. I highly recommend the use of champignon mushrooms to achieve and maintain gut health in dogs. My ideal formula for establishing and maintaining great gut health would include:

- Probiotic blend (1 billion CFUs per serving): to help digest food into "fuel," promote a calm, happy mood, and support a healthy immune system.
- Plaque-fighting Icelandic kelp (*Ascophyllum nodosum*): to improve oral health, promote better-smelling breath, and support coat and skin.
- Odor-reducing Champex: derived from champignon mushrooms, this extract can support probiotic growth and dramatically reduce body odor and smelly poops.
- Digestive enzymes: to ease digestion, promote more solid poops, and support skin and coat health.
- Prebiotic blend (fructooligosaccharides): prebiotic fiber to help support the growth of probiotics.

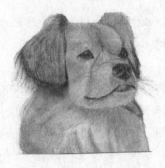

6

OTHER REMARKABLE
THERAPIES

*The next wave of medical advances will be when
we come to recognize the body as an energetic system.*
—LISA OZ

Many years ago, one of my employees gave me a fascinating gift, a medical textbook published by the New York University College of Medicine in the 1890s. She bought it at a garage sale for $1. Opening the book, I was surprised to see that the "drugs" commonly used to treat a variety of ailments over a century ago were different species and parts of plants and vegetables.

Fast-forward to modern-day medical therapy. Many of the pills used in current veterinary practice are colorful—red, magenta, yellow, and black. Do you think the dog or cat in your life cares what the color of these pills are? (No, dogs and cats couldn't care less—their color perception is limited.)

Are the dyes used to color the pills free of side effects? (No, they often have toxic effects.)[1] The designs and colors of today's pills are carefully engineered to appeal to pet *parents*. It's all about *marketing,* not so much *therapeutics.*

My life's work has been to try to get back to more natural therapies, therapies that have been on this planet for thousands of years. As we have seen in the preceding chapters, just feeding your animal companions high-quality food and the right nutraceuticals can go a long way to keep them in good health.

Beyond the power of feeding our animal companions the right food and nutraceutical supplements, however, a variety of cutting-edge therapies are currently in use, with others in research and just over the horizon. Some you may be familiar with, and others not.

In this chapter, I explore the most promising of these remarkable therapies, including the administration of high-dose intravenous vitamin C as an effective treatment for cancer; stem cell therapy to treat arthritis and ligament, tendon, kidney, and other problems; MagnaWave / pulsed electromagnetic field (PEMF) therapy to treat arthritis, injuries, and spinal and neurological ailments—even cancer—and more. Let's dive right in!

HIGH-DOSE VITAMIN C

Vitamin C (also called L-ascorbic acid or ascorbate) is a nutrient that acts as an antioxidant at typical dietary and supplement doses. However, when given at high doses intravenously, vitamin C becomes a pro-oxidant. Both of these functions of vitamin C aim to reduce oxidative stress at the cellular level in the body, but by different methods.

First, what is oxidative stress? *Oxidative stress* is an important function in the body to help with healing by creating inflammation. However, if unchecked because of a weak immune system, oxidative stress creates excessive inflammation and ultimately disease. Every disease process has at its source oxidative stress.

Let me say that again—*slowly*.

Every disease process has at its source oxidative stress.

At high doses given directly into the bloodstream, vitamin C has a unique ability to both prevent oxidative stress and reverse the damage done by it.[2] The antioxidant function of vitamin C aids the immune system in preventing and fighting disease by reducing oxidative stress through the immune system. Synergistically, the pro-oxidant function of vitamin C achieved only at high doses directly reduces oxidative stress inside diseased cells in the body. At high doses, both the antioxidant and pro-oxidant function of vitamin C is achieved, and healing therefore takes place at multiple levels.

Humans must obtain vitamin C from food or dietary supplements since it cannot be made in the body. Most companion animals, on the other hand, are able to synthesize vitamin C on their own if they're healthy—and *healthy* is the key word. In general, I do not like giving vitamin C to a healthy dog or cat because it could inhibit their natural production, and we don't want to do that. But vitamin C has become so successful—especially at high doses—because of our practices of ill health over the generations. Many of these animals that should be making their own vitamin C have lost that ability.

High-dose vitamin C has been studied as a treatment for patients with cancer since the 1970s. A Scottish surgeon named Ewan Cameron worked with Nobel Prize–winning chemist Linus Pauling to study the possible benefits of vitamin C therapy in clinical trials of cancer patients in the late 1970s and early 1980s. In their groundbreaking study, one hundred terminal cancer patients received supplemental ascorbate (vitamin C). Their outcomes were compared with those of one thousand "similar patients treated identically, but who received no supplemental ascorbate." According to Cameron and Pauling, the mean survival time was "more than 4.2 times as great for the ascorbate subjects (more than 210 days) as for the controls (50 days)."[3]

My colleague Dr. George Zabrecky introduced me to the work of Dr. Hugh Riordan, who with benefactor Olive Garvey founded the Riordan Clinic in Wichita, Kansas, in 1975. The most notable body of work from Dr. Riordan is on the administration of megadoses of vitamins to human patients—specifically vitamin C (fifty grams and higher)—and the positive effect this has on many chronic illnesses. A follower of Linus Pauling, Dr. Riordan based his vitamin C protocol in part on the findings of the noted Nobel Prize–winning chemist.

Dr. Riordan authored four books, three of which deal with "medical mavericks"—a subject that he found quite interesting, probably because he himself was a maverick about nutrition and medicine. Dr. Riordan also authored more than seventy-nine medical-journal articles and papers, many of which were published in peer-reviewed journals. The vast majority of his papers dealt with the benefits of vitamin C. Today, the Riordan Clinic continues to be at the forefront of research on high-dose intravenous vitamin C therapy. In addition, they host an annual symposium on IV vitamin C for medical doctors.

According to the clinic, the Riordan IVC protocol addresses cancer in a comprehensive way, leading to the following outcomes:

- Boosts immunity (to prevent secondary infections)
- Stimulates collagen formation (to wall off tumors)
- Inhibits hyaluronidase (to retard metastasis)
- Relieves cellular hypoxia / restores aerobic metabolism
- Restores mitochondrial functioning, including apoptosis
- Inhibits angiogenesis and reduces tumor nutrient supply
- Corrects scurvy in cancer patients (less fatigue)
- Is immune activating (fights underlying infections)
- Supports detoxification systems in the body
- Relieves pain and promotes well-being
- Potentiates chemotherapy and radiation
- Reduces side effects and toxicity of conventional therapy[4]

As you can see, this is pretty much like having all of your cake and getting to eat it, too.

My brother and I treated over a dozen cats with leukemia years ago using high doses of vitamin C. We observed:

- Not only were these terminal cats getting better, but several of the National Veterinary Laboratory feline leukemia (FeLV) tests reverted from positive to negative, which was unheard of and blew our minds.

- The blood level of vitamin C reached is just as important as the amount administered. If you give a thirty-pound dog twenty grams of vitamin C over twenty-four hours, it probably won't kill cancer cells. However, if you give that same dose over three hours, it will.
- Vitamin C creates high osmolarity in the blood, which increases the chances of its being pushed into tissues.
- Vitamin C has both an immediate and a long-term effect.

High-dose vitamin C may be given by intravenous (IV) infusion (through a vein into the bloodstream) or orally (taken by mouth). However, vitamin C taken intravenously can reach much higher levels in the blood than when the same amount is taken by mouth. This is in part because large amounts of vitamin C given orally usually instigate diarrhea. The lining of the intestine can become seriously inflamed as a result of direct contact with the vitamin.

Normally, diarrhea is actually a good sign when we're administering vitamin C intravenously. It shows that the vitamin C has caused a detoxification of the body through the liver, which then uses in part the intestines as its dumping ground. After we help a companion animal regain his good health, some of our clients will ask if they can administer an ongoing oral dose of vitamin C themselves. They can, but not at high doses. If you administer an oral dose of vitamin C anywhere near the high doses we give intravenously, the dog or cat will experience intense diarrhea. If the diarrhea is intense enough for long enough, the patient may require medical supervision. So, we warn our clients not to try to do high doses themselves at home.

To give you an idea of the scale of what I'm talking about, when my brother and I started exploring treatment of feline leukemia–positive cats with high doses of vitamin C, we would buy a kilogram—2.2 pounds—of sodium ascorbate powder (a mineral salt of ascorbic acid, which is vitamin C) at a time. We were taking two or three teaspoons of the sodium ascorbate powder (one teaspoon equaled about four thousand milligrams), dissolving it in some IV fluid, and giving it to a feline patient intravenously. And as I already mentioned, we saw remarkable results.

Today, high-dose IV vitamin C therapy is a routine treatment at Smith Ridge Veterinary Center. For that I have to give a tip of the hat to my colleague Dr. Jacqueline Ruskin, who took hold of the idea, studied it deeply, and developed highly effective treatment protocols. She is also a contributor to this section. The lives of many companion animals have been improved—and even saved—as a result of Dr. Ruskin's work in this area. In those days, if word had gotten out that we were doing this, our licenses wouldn't have had a chance of surviving the week.

According to the Siteman Cancer Center, high doses of vitamin C have been found by researchers to slow the growth and spread of prostate, pancreatic, liver, colon, and other types of cancer cells. In addition, the Siteman Cancer Center says that when vitamin C and certain anticancer therapies are combined, research has found that the effect is enhanced. On the other hand, certain forms of vitamin C have been found by researchers to make chemotherapy less effective.[5] That is why I rarely recommend doing them together because vitamin C is a powerful detoxifier. When an animal is on chemo—a highly toxic substance—you don't want to flush it out or inactivate it with vitamin C.

While high-dose IV vitamin C has not been approved by the FDA to treat cancer or other medical conditions in humans, it is used by medical doctors, naturopaths, and on-cologists around the globe—and by integrative veterinarians, especially the ones at Smith Ridge Veterinary Center—for cancer and other diseases. The FDA does not regulate the use of oral or intravenous vitamin C in pets. In chapter 11, I'll talk about the potential benefits of IV vitamin C that were revealed during the COVID-19 global pandemic.

At Smith Ridge, we have treated thousands of animals with IV vitamin C and have seen almost as many incredible results. Not only have our patients experienced tumor regres-sion, but also a return of appetite and life force. Interestingly enough, so many of their other chronic conditions, such as arthritis, skin disease, and many more were also improved. So, now we don't use this intravenous therapy just for can-cer patients, but also for many other chronic, nonresponsive medical conditions.

Because of how many cases we have treated that returned home better, we have been asked by many attending vet-erinarians around the country to share our protocol for IV vitamin C. Our consistent answer is that, unfortunately, we don't have a protocol. All of our patients are treated individ-ually depending on their diagnosis, overall condition, age, weight, blood results, ability to acclimate, and other factors. Two dogs of similar weight and diagnosis can and often do receive totally different amounts of vitamin C over their typically three-day course of therapy.

ASK DR. MARTY

Q: A lot of veterinarians today call themselves integrative or holistic, but how do you really know? How can I find a good integrative veterinarian?

A: I have a few recommendations. First, I along with most other reputable integrative veterinarians belong to the American Holistic Veterinary Medical Association. If you go to their website (ahvma.org), you can use their "Find a Vet" search function to look for an integrative veterinarian near you. You can search by practice type (for example, small animal, feline only, equine, farm, avian, and so on), by modalities (acupuncture, homeopathy, ozone therapy, Chinese herbs, and so on), and by state or province.

Second, do searches on Google and online business-directory services such as Yelp.com. Both Google and Yelp provide user ratings and reviews, which can be helpful in your search. Just be aware that some businesses pay people to get a good review, and some good businesses can receive bad reviews when they don't deserve it. The old saying caveat emptor definitely applies.

Third, ask around. If you take your dog to a dog park for exercise or playtime, or if you have friends or relatives with dogs or cats, ask other pet parents. Go to a local health food store and ask whom they recommend. Good veterinarians will over time develop good reputations, and health food stores can be a great source of information. When you ask, someone will chime in, "Oh—go see Dr. Smith—she's *awesome.*" Or "I wouldn't take my dead cat to see Dr. So-and-So." Pet parents who love and care for their animal companions usually know who the best veterinarians are in the area, whether they're integrative or not.

If you don't live close to a large city, you may have to travel out of your area to get the best care. A few years ago, we did a survey at Smith Ridge Veterinary Center over several weeks to see where most of our patients came from. To our surprise, the average client that came specifically to see me was 590 miles away from our clinic. You don't necessarily have to travel to get care from a veterinarian whose practice is far from your home. We have helped literally thousands and thousands of patients over the years by doing phone consults, including their local veterinarian in the loop for diagnosis and medical advice.

We have seen some remarkable results in animals that came to Smith Ridge with terminal illnesses. When we sent them back home after their treatments, they were getting better. But when veterinarians tried to replicate our approach, at times it was not as effective as what we were doing at Smith Ridge, only because we had so much experience patient by patient. If you decide to get intravenous vitamin C therapy for your companion animal, make sure it's done at a facility that is well experienced in its use.

STEM CELL THERAPY

Stem cells are a special type of cell in humans, dogs, cats, and other organisms that are not differentiated—that is, they have not yet "decided" what kind of cell they will be in the body. They are also *pluripotent*, meaning they have the potential to develop into any of the more than 220 cell types in the adult body—for example, red skeletal-muscle cells, white blood cells, spinal nerve cells, and so forth. Humans and animals are generally considered to have two kinds of stem cells: *embryonic* (derived from preimplantation embryos) and *non-embryonic* (also known as *somatic* or *adult* stem cells).

The big excitement around stem cells is their ability in so many cases to maintain, replenish, and repair damaged or depleted cells. A relatively new field, *regenerative medicine,* is the replacing or regenerating of cells, tissues, or organs using a variety of different methods. Regenerative medicine has the same potential to help our animal companions as it does humans. According to the FDA:

In the fast-growing field of veterinary regenerative medicine, cellular materials—such as living cells, serum, or other products derived from cells—are used in animals with the hope of repairing diseased or damaged tissues or organs. For example, in a horse with tendonitis, the damaged tendon may heal with scar tissue that isn't as strong or elastic as the original tendon before it was damaged. The goal is to transplant living cells into the injured tendon, hopefully stimulating it to regenerate and heal. Veterinary regenerative medicine is an active area of research for developing new therapies for animals.[6]

Because of their unique properties, stem cells are one of the most promising avenues for the pursuit of regenerative medicine. The pioneer in the use of stem cell therapy in dogs, cats, and horses is VetStem Biopharma (www.vetstem.com), founded by its current CEO, Dr. Bob Harman, in 2002. More than fourteen thousand animals have been treated since then.

The VetStem procedure works like this: A veterinarian collects a small amount of fat from your dog, cat, or horse under local or general anesthesia. The fat is shipped overnight via FedEx to the VetStem laboratory near San Diego for processing, isolating, and concentrating of stem cells. The cells are then returned to the veterinarian for implantation at the site of the injury or intravenously within forty-eight hours of collection.

VetStem is currently treating a variety of conditions using stem cells. In dogs and cats, this includes osteoarthritis, orthopedic soft-tissue injuries, polyarthritis, and fractures. According to the company's data, at thirty, sixty, and ninety days post–stem cell treatment, more than 80 percent of dogs with orthopedic conditions showed an improved quality of life according to owners and veterinarians.[7] In addition, 81 percent of older dogs (nine to eighteen years old) with osteoarthritis showed an improved quality of life, and 63 percent did not have to be re-treated in the first year.[8] Those are some pretty remarkable results.

Another company that's been on my radar screen for some time is MediVet Biologics in Kentucky (www.medivetbiologics

.com). The company's mission is "to offer innovative, safe and effective biologic treatments in regenerative medicine & oncology solutions, to assist millions of animals needlessly suffering in pain." The company uses an approach called *autologous stem cell therapy* (the same as VetStem) because the source of the cells is the patient's own body. This way, there are no ethical or moral issues as with stem cells derived from embryonic and other sources.

MediVet has treated a variety of conditions with its stem cell therapy, including osteoarthritis (hip dysplasia, degenerative joint disease, calcifications, common degeneration, and inflammation) and soft-tissue injuries. In addition, the company treats other cases under "compassionate use," including degenerative myelopathy, feline gingivitis, end-stage renal disease, allergies, inflammatory bowel disease, spine trauma, and more. I am especially excited by the early evidence for treatment in end-stage renal disease, allergies, and inflammatory bowel disease.

The real beauty of the MediVet protocol is that the company brings the equipment and training into the veterinarian's facility. This makes harvesting the fat; processing, isolating, and concentrating stem cells; and injecting them into the dog, cat, or equine patient possible in the same day.

More important, does it work? According to MediVet, in one study 155 dogs suffering from moderate to severe osteoarthritis were treated with the company's stem cell therapy. At the end of ninety days, 99 percent of the dogs showed improvements in at least one of the three analyzed categories: lameness, range of motion, and pain.[9]

This phenomenal result clearly demonstrates the tremendous potential for the use of stem cell therapy in our animal companions. Osteoarthritis is just the tip of the iceberg for conditions that may one day be treated using stem cells. Research has been conducted with stem cells in veterinary medicine to see if they can successfully treat animals with cancer, diabetes, heart disease, immune disorders, loss of bladder control, and even kidney failure. The possibilities seem endless. Note, however, that using stem cells to treat cancer is *not* recommended because in some cases it can instigate further cancer growth.

Another popular aspect of regenerative medicine associated with stem cell therapy is called platelet-rich plasma or PRP. Plasma is the liquid fraction of whole blood, and *platelets* or *thrombocytes* are the cells that swim in the plasma and play a key role in healing. When you cut your finger, these platelets cause your blood to clot and your wound to stop bleeding. They then stimulate and increase the number of reparative cells produced by the body, including the recruitment of stem cells. Being chock-full of growth factors themselves, once activated, platelets have a direct effect on wound healing.

Compared to stem cell injections, PRP injections are a shorter-term solution to inflammation and injuries of joints, tendons, ligaments, and even muscles. With the proper equipment and kits, veterinarians can do this procedure right in their own clinics.

While research in stem cell therapy for dogs and cats is still in its infancy, and access and cost are currently barriers for those who want to try it, I believe that it will one day have a remarkable impact on the lives of many millions of animal companions. I recommend that every pet parent keep an eye on progress in this emerging and fast-changing veterinary medical field.

A KENTUCKY COLONEL

Dr. Bob Harman, founder of VetStem, and I became good friends years ago.

One day, I received an email from Bob—a VIP client had contacted him about some problems with his dog. Bob wanted to work on the dog, the dog and client lived on the East Coast, and Bob didn't want to proceed unless I got involved. I was busy at the time, and I didn't need another VIP client. I pushed Bob's request to the back burner.

Weeks passed. One Monday, however, I looked at my schedule for the week and noticed that I didn't have anything booked for Tuesday, which was my usual day to do surgeries. So, I thought, "You know what? I'll call this client that Bob wants to send me." I called the guy and he told me about his thirteen-year-old French poodle, Edelweiss—Edel, for short. The dog had severe cataracts and was blind.

Edel had already been examined by one of the top veterinary ophthalmologists in the country. He told the client that removing the cataracts would be like taking the lens cap off a camera that has no film—in addition to cataracts, Edel also had retinal atrophy. So even if the cataracts were removed, Edel's vision would not be restored.

The client's wife had been undergoing successful stem cell therapy in South America. Because she responded so well to the therapy, they started looking for someone in the United States doing stem cell therapy with animals. They found Bob Harman—he was the only one in the United States at the time who was FDA approved to do this type of therapy. The client and Dr. Harman spoke and decided together to collect stem cells from Edel, fly over to Israel, and get a renowned vet there to inject the cells into Edel's eyes—hopefully enabling them to regenerate. Again, Dr. Harman didn't want to work with this client unless I was involved.

During my call with the client, I told him that I had time to examine Edelweiss on Tuesday and asked, "Is there any way you can bring Edelweiss to Smith Ridge?"

"I have my own jet airplane," he replied, "so I'll be there."

Tuesday morning, the client walked through the door of Smith Ridge with Edel. It was John Hendrickson, a tennis pro who used to teach at the Nick Bollettieri / IMG Tennis Academy outside Bradenton, Florida.

After talking about Edelweiss's medical issues for a while, I decided to check with a talented veterinary ophthalmologist in the area, Dr. Chuck Stuhr. He had removed the cataracts from my dog Nina with great success. I called him up and explained John Hendrickson's plan to take Edel to Israel to have stem cells injected into her eyes.

"The veterinarian in Israel you're talking about is a colleague of mine," Chuck said. "Look, you don't have to fly this dog to Israel—I'll inject her eyes."

"Great!" I said. "I'll be in touch."

I explained to John that Dr. Harman could process Edel's stem cells, then the local ophthalmologist would inject them.

"But," I continued, "I work on more than just the symptoms. Let's get Edel healthy."

"Let's go for it," John replied.

I collected a blood sample from Edel, and I gave her an injection of homeopathic retina and homeopathic eyeball—organ-specific homeopathic remedies that we were able, at the time, to import from Germany. Then John and Edel flew back home on their jet.

Nineteen hours later, I received an email from John:

> Dear Dr. Goldstein,
> Thank you very much for seeing us yesterday. Edel is already responding well to the new therapy. She is now able to see us from across the room, and her bad cataract is already shrinking. Thank you, thank you. Marylou and I are VERY grateful.
> I've already called Mrs. Schwartz [husband Barry was the CEO of Calvin Klein] and told them how great you are, and to meet you someday.

Edel needed more of these homeopathic injections, so a week later, my family and I hopped in our minivan and we drove up to the Vanderbilt estate in Saratoga, where Edel lived with John and his wife, Marylou Whitney. Edel could see, and she ended up not getting the stem cell injections into her eyes. As we were all talking about Edel, John and I spoke about the possibility of my giving two lectures in Kentucky—one specifically for veterinarians, and one for the public. John decided to sponsor the lectures and we made plans to get them set up.

A few months later, I flew to Kentucky where I lectured to veterinarians for two and a half hours, and to the public for three hours. During one of those lectures, the governor of Kentucky came up onstage and gave me a certificate. The certificate officially named me a Kentucky Colonel—the highest title bestowed by the Kentucky governor—which has been awarded to all sorts of notable people, including Muhammad Ali, Shirley Temple, Tiger Woods, Betty White, Paul McCartney, and many others. It now hangs proudly on my office wall.

Thank you, Edelweiss! Thank you for the wonders of homeopathy!

ASK DR. MARTY

Q: I'm sure you have experienced many remarkable changes in the medical field over your nearly five-decade career. How do you feel advancements in technology have influenced these changes?

A: You're right—the medical field has gone through some remarkable changes over the past five decades. I'm impressed by, and at times in awe of, the many technological wonders that exist today. For example, advances in imaging allow us to view and diagnose any part of a dog's or a cat's body with incredible accuracy down to a millimeter. This is a staggering change from the old-fashioned X-rays we had to develop by hand and work with when I graduated from veterinary school in the 1970s. The ability to tightly focus a beam of radiation to zap a patient's brain tumor with minimal damage to the surrounding normal tissue is also impressive. But, that said, we humans still don't come close to the amazing level of creation and intelligence of Mother Nature herself. This is why some of the most profoundly effective methods of healing, such as acupuncture and herbs—which are thousands of years old and not technologically advanced—work so well even today. It's because they align with natural healing pathways instead of overpowering them with science.

FECAL TRANSPLANTS

Have you ever heard the saying "Shit happens"? I'll bet you have. You may even have adopted these two simple words as a life philosophy. As you know from personal experience, every animal on the face of this earth eats food and occasionally other things, and every animal on the face of this earth poops out the digested remains of all that stuff it ate. This cycle fuels our bodies and keeps us and our animal companions alive and well.

But there's more to poop than just the remains of whatever food and other stuff an animal ate.

Poop contains a fragrant mix of water, fiber, bacteria, fungi, viruses, mucus, and other random things. In the case of a dog, these random things might include grass, bits of bone, pieces of torn-apart tennis balls, tapeworms, roundworms, hookworms, and more. One gram of dog poop typically contains on average 23 million fecal coliform bacteria.[10]

Poop is a reflection of the *microbiome*—the collection of microbes that live in the gut, skin, respiratory tract, ears, and mouth of a dog, cat, or other creature, but mostly in the gut. (Research shows that dogs and their pet parents who live together in the same household share similar microbiomes.)[11]

According to *Dogs Naturally Magazine,* your dog's microbiome serves five key functions:

- **Protection against pathogens.** The good bacteria and other microbes in the microbiome can outnumber bad bacteria and even secrete chemicals that protect from the harmful effects of viruses, fungi, and bad bacteria.
- **Forms a protective barrier.** The microbiome can keep toxins from moving deeper into the dog's body while defending against drugs, allergens, and carcinogens.
- **Feeds your dog.** Your dog's microbiome produces enzymes that aid digestion as well as vitamins (particularly B vitamins) and short-chain fatty acids.
- **Affects your dog's mood.** The brain communicates with the microbiome through something called the gut-brain axis—"the constant bidirectional communication between the gastrointestinal tract and the brain." Research indicates that the microbes in the gut of your dog or cat can have a direct effect on brain biochemistry and behavior.[12]
- **Is a critical part of the immune system.** A dog's intestinal tract is lined with a mucous membrane called gut-associated lymphoid tissue, or GALT for short. GALT is chock-full of immune cells, including lymphocytes, and T and B cells, and is thought to comprise approximately 90 percent of a dog's immune system.[13]

The microbiome serves the same function in cats, humans, and other animals as well.

But what happens when gastrointestinal systems get out of whack, and the normal, good bacteria that live there are damaged or destroyed by drugs, chemicals in the environment, or other trauma? The microbiome can suffer, with good microbes dying off and bad microbes taking over. This can cause all sorts of problems for dogs and cats, including inflammatory bowel disease, diabetes, parasites, obesity, allergies, mood disorders, autoimmune issues, and perhaps even cancer.[14]

So, what can be done to restore a microbiome to good health? One unique approach is called *fecal microbiota transplant*, or FMT. In this procedure poop from a healthy dog, cat, or human is placed into an infected dog, cat, or human. I have known Dr. Margo Roman of Main Street Animal Services of Hopkinton (MASH) in Hopkinton, Massachusetts, for many years. She was a classmate of mine in the acupuncture class I attended in the mid-seventies to get certified by the International Veterinary Acupuncture Society. We always sat together, and we've been good friends and colleagues ever since.

According to Dr. Roman, the fecal transplant procedure— which she calls *microbiome restorative therapy*, or MBRT— does more than just replace the bacteria in the gut. Because the gut plays such a vital role in immune response, FMT/MBRT has the ability to "start to rebuild that immune system from the inside."[15]

In an interview with Dr. Karen Becker, Dr. Roman explained how she first learned about MBRT:

I read an article about a physician who had a woman he was treating for *Clostridium difficile* (*C. diff*). *Clostridium difficile* actually kills about fourteen thousand people in the United States a year. It's really a very serious issue. They think that three hundred thousand people in the United States get it, and over a million probably get it but they're not documented. The woman was dying, and she was down to like eighty pounds. He basically took the husband's feces, put it in a blender, put it through a nasogastric tube (NG tube), and gave it to the wife. Within two days, she was having normal bowel movements and completely recovered. He did like 120 cases with 97 percent success with one treatment.[16]

While probiotics have their place as a nutraceutical, according to Dr. Roman, they aren't particularly effective when an entire microbiome is compromised. Human beings have on the order of 100 trillion microbes within them, which comprise five hundred species and thousands of subspecies. No probiotic currently available even begins to make a dent in that rich intestinal flora.

After reading the article about the physician who used MBRT to treat a patient infected by *Clostridium difficile*, Dr. Roman committed to one day trying the technique on a sick dog. Her opportunity came with Stovin, an emaciated dog brought to her with severe gastrointestinal problems and Addison's disease. The dog's parent had already spent more than $16,000 to treat the dog at an animal medical center. Says Dr. Roman, "I gave him the ozone, the acupuncture, and the fecal transplant, and he completely recovered. You would not even know his picture before and after . . . he doesn't look like the same dog."[17]

In another case, Dr. Roman treated a cat that presented with severe atopic dermatitis. The cat had scabs on his face, and he was angry and miserable. Explains Dr. Roman, "We gave him a fecal transplant from my cat, Trapper, who was raised on a raw diet and who didn't get neutered until he was a year old."[18] Within a week after the treatment, the cat's coat had started to come back in, and he was happy and no longer scratching himself.

As an adjunct to MBRT, Dr. Roman has also pioneered treatment with medical ozone. According to Dr. Roman, the amount of CO_2 increases in tissue as a result of inflammation, swelling, infection, bruising, and cancer. By administering medical ozone, oxygen is brought into the tissue, the excess CO_2 is displaced, and inflammation, infection, and bruising are decreased.

While fecal microbiota transplant might seem counterintuitive—introducing the poop from a healthy dog or cat to one that is sick—it makes perfect sense. You're restoring what's missing in the sick animal's microbiome, which enables it to overcome the bad microbes that have taken hold and to become healthy once again. It's a simple but extremely powerful procedure. It warms my heart to see that a procedure—which could be considered by some to be in the realm of "holistic quackery"—is scientifically accepted by esteemed institutions such as Johns Hopkins and Memorial Sloan Kettering Cancer Center.[19]

PULSED ELECTROMAGNETIC
FIELD THERAPY

Pulsed electromagnetic field (PEMF) therapy is the use of pulsed magnetic fields created by moving electrical charges to treat humans and dogs, cats, horses, and other animals. The use of electrical stimulation to induce healing in humans (specifically, of an unconsolidated fracture of the tibia by John Birch, a London surgeon, in 1812) was first described in an 1841 paper by Edward Hartshorne.[20] However, using PEMF to treat companion animals is relatively recent. I was introduced to the wonders of this therapy in a roundabout way.

I have been friends for many years with Cindy Meehl, creator and director of *The Dog Doc*—the documentary film featuring me and my life's work. Years ago, Cindy kept bugging me that I needed to check in with a husband-and-wife team of chiropractors in Connecticut—Dave and Wendy—who were using a technology called MagnaWave to treat horses and dogs in addition to their human patients. I called their office, and they told me they were leaving the next day to treat horses for several months down in Wellington, Florida.

Wellington is a major equestrian center, sometimes called the horse capital of America. During the town's Winter Equestrian Festival, scheduled from January to April every year, the country's best horses and riders compete for $9 million in prize money. Competitors have included the daughters of Steve Jobs, Bill Gates, Michael Bloomberg, Bruce

Springsteen, Steven Spielberg, Tom Selleck, Jerry Seinfeld, Madonna, and Lorne Michaels, and other horse-loving celebrities who have lived in the area during the festival and beyond.[21]

Dave and Wendy invited me to come over that night, before they left for Florida. So I drove over to their place in Redding, Connecticut. They greeted me at the door, and when I walked in, a relatively young man—probably in his late twenties—was lying on a table on top of a full-length body mat that was attached by heavy wire cables to a forty-pound boxlike device on wheels. He was in the middle of a MagnaWave treatment for irritable bowel syndrome. I remember sitting down on a chair to watch the treatment proceed. I was at his body level, and as I watched, his abdomen pulsed up and down in concert with the energy this machine was delivering to the mat on which he was lying. At one point he said to Wendy, "Can you turn it down a little? It's a little bit uncomfortable."

After the treatment, he got off the table and said, "Oh my God—my abdomen feels so much better!"

After he left, Wendy looked at me. "Do you want to try this machine?"

"Absolutely." I explained that, when I was younger, I had had arthritis and bursitis of my left shoulder, and it flared up every once in a while. So, I lay my entire body down on the mat, and they turned on the machine—gradually increasing the power, up and up and up. I started to feel it pulse in my shoulder.

They treated me for ten minutes, and my shoulder felt better than it had felt in the previous twenty years. My mind was blown. So much so that I begged them not to go to Florida: "Please don't go. I need more of this."

But then I looked at them and said, "Wait a minute. I was on the exact same mat as the young man with irritable bowel syndrome, and his abdomen pulsed when you were treating him. *My* abdomen didn't pulse—just my shoulder—and you turned the machine's power control knob quite high. How does it do that?"

Wendy replied, "Because it knows"—meaning the Magna-Wave machine has the ability to also be diagnostic of where disease exists in the body.

Sometime later, a client of mine, Steve (Elsa's pet parent, whom we'll talk about in chapter 7), told me that his friend had a MagnaWave machine. That got my attention. The friend had done well in business and retired. He and his fiancée started a dog boarding and grooming business called Fetch near the Brooklyn–Battery Tunnel in Manhattan. I called the guy and said, "My name is Dr. Marty."

"Oh, I know who you are. Steve doesn't stop raving about you."

After chatting a bit, I asked about the machine: "Steve told me that you've got a machine you bought a while ago, and it's possibly a MagnaWave. Is that what you've got?"

"Yeah, that's what I have. It's been sitting in my closet for a year."

My heart skipped a beat or two. "Can I borrow it?"

"Absolutely."

So, I drove down, we had dinner, and I told him I would help promote his store and come down there and lecture for him. He loaned me the MagnaWave to try out. I brought it back to Smith Ridge and started to use it—first on myself and some of my staff, and then we started treating animals with it. After about nine months, the guy who owned the MagnaWave asked if I was interested in buying the machine and keeping it. I said yes, and it's still the one we use at Smith Ridge today.

During all this, I met Pat Ziemer. I had become friends with Wendy and Dave, the chiropractors who introduced me to MagnaWave, and after I bought my own machine—now secondhand—I called to tell them the good news. They suggested that I get the machine serviced and gave me Pat's name and number. I called Pat—he knew the model I had because he had originally sold it. I was headed to Boston to speak about nutraceuticals at a weekend seminar on rehabilitation put on by the University of Tennessee College of Veterinary Medicine. I told Pat that I planned to devote part of my talk to the MagnaWave.

Pat immediately said, "I'm flying in to meet you."

So, he flew to Boston to meet me. He brought his Magna-Wave and gave it to me, and I gave him my MagnaWave to get serviced. I asked him how he found out about this therapy. He told me that he had formerly had a business selling and leasing private jets. After 9/11 in 2001, his business did not survive. He was living in Louisville, Kentucky, at the time, so to make a living, he started selling low-voltage PEMF equipment and hyaluronic acid supplements for horses, especially at Churchill Downs.

Pat and his wife, Debi, went to a health-and-wellness convention—Debi had three herniated discs in her neck and an ascending aortic aneurysm. Because of the herniated discs, she had for years experienced limited mobility and constant pain. A high-voltage PEMF company was giving demonstrations of the version of their machine for humans at the convention—treating anyone who was interested. That's how they sold their machines. Pat's wife had a demonstration treatment and felt great afterward.

The next day, as they were driving back to Louisville after the convention, Pat asked her what she thought about the machine. She replied, "I bought it!" Pat says that he almost drove off the road. Months later, Pat's wife went back to her cardiologist, who said that during his entire career, he had never seen an aneurysm shrink. Hers did.

At Churchill Downs, Pat started treating horses with PEMF with great success. But his machine was a smaller, more exposed tabletop unit for people, and the horses were yanking it around—potentially damaging it. Pat contacted the manufacturer to see if they could make a more durable model. The company replied, "Will you help us do that?" Pat did just that, and he created the MagnaWave company.

Every single year when I introduce MagnaWave in my talks, I have a slide in my PowerPoint presentation of the chamber in the starship *Enterprise* you would enter if you got sick or had any ailment, and a beam of light would go through your body, and you'd be well again. That to me is the promise of pulsed electromagnetic field therapy and MagnaWave. This remarkable technology has changed countless lives for the better—including animal companions *and* their pet parents. As Dr. Oz said about MagnaWave, "Today we are changing the future of medicine and pain relief."[22]

PULSED ELECTROMAGNETIC FIELD THERAPY

by Pat Ziemer

Founder and CEO, MagnaWave[23]

Since early 2002, I have been utilizing pulsed electromagnetic field (PEMF) therapy in the treatment of large and small animals as well as humans. While I am neither a doctor nor a veterinarian, my postcollege studies included microbiology and pathology, and I have been a practicing EMT. Over these years, I have continually been learning, researching, and applying the principles of this remarkably powerful therapy.

In 2008, two equine and human chiropractic practitioners who use MagnaWave PEMF turned Dr. Marty on to the potential benefits and uses of the therapy. Naturally, Dr. Marty wanted to know the complete background, so my associates suggested that he give me a call. He did just that, and we initially talked for nearly two hours about the therapy and its value and processes. Since that time, we have become close friends and associates in research, application, understanding, and education for those new to the world of PEMF therapy.

Inflammation is the number one cause of pain in the body. The use of pulsed electromagnetic fields provides a means to reduce inflammation and thereby reduce and relieve pain. The primary function is to improve oxygenation and improve blood flow in the body.

Magnetic fields affect the charge of the cell membrane, which opens up the cells' membrane channels. These channels are like the doors and windows of a house for airflow and circulation. By opening cell channels, nutrients are easily absorbed by the cell and waste easily eliminated. The process helps to rebalance and restore optimum cell function. If you continually utilize PEMF to restore cells, they will all work more efficiently. By using PEMF for restoring or maintaining cellular function, you will, in turn, repair or maintain organ function, allowing the entire body to function better and maintain wellness.

We also know that the body ages, and that an essential part of slowing aging is to keep the function of every individual cell at an optimal level. A by-product of this cellular rejuvenation provided by MagnaWave PEMF is the feeling of well-being from maintaining optimum cellular health. This sense of well-being becomes the basis for excellent results for many indications by providing relief from pain that leads to healing.

A new angle on stress, depression, anxiety, arthritis, and other disease manifestations is the inflammation connection. Recent studies have shown how the immune system and inflammation play a role in the development of these indications. They also show that targeting specific elements of the inflammatory process can be useful in treating or preventing these and other disorders. Various drugs and medications are typically given to fight the body's inflammation processes. The use of MagnaWave PEMF has demonstrated the promise of a drug-free method of fighting the damaging effects of inflammation as a part of disease.

The PEMF modality has gained FDA clearance for uses in humans that include non-union fractures (where the two parts do not heal or knit to each other), depression, autism, incontinence, and brain tumors. The PEMF modality is regularly used to improve any indication that could benefit from improved oxygenation and inflammation reduction. The list of positive-result uses is long and growing and includes everything from arthritis to stress-related diseases and speedier recovery.

Here's one more aspect of PEMF therapy worth mentioning: When I was doing my research, I found an article about people with bone tumors. They were intravenously administered a strong chemotherapeutic called cisplatin. The uptake of this drug in the tumor was measured to be 17 percent. Later on, in the same patient, the same medication and same dose were given, but the area of the tumor was treated with PEMF. The uptake of cisplatin increased to 37 percent.

At one of the MagnaWave annual conferences in Lexington, Kentucky, which I attend and lecture at every June, a presenter offered science-based evidence that PEMF can increase absorption of a medicinal substance by 200 percent—a remarkable result. I feel that, on the human side, this is our answer—our ray of hope—for many deep-seated conditions such as ALS, Parkinson's, Alzheimer's, MS, and so on.

HYPERTHERMIA

In my first book, I shared an incredible case of a boxer named Ginger who, in the final stages of eliminating leukemia and lymph cancer from her body, ran a fever of at least 107°. This case is so astounding that, despite its being decades old, I still present it when I lecture to veterinarians and professionals. Although Ginger's body did this on its own, hyperthermia can be administered in several ways, either as a primary treatment or to enhance other therapies.

According to the hyperthermia fact sheet published by the National Cancer Institute, "Research has shown that high temperatures can damage and kill cancer cells, usually with minimal injury to normal tissues. By killing cancer cells and damaging proteins and structures within cells, hyperthermia may shrink tumors."[24]

In the hypothalamus of the brain is a temperature regulation (thermoregulation) center—it's what keeps our internal temperature stable when the temperature outside varies. So, when I go soak myself in a 185° sauna or go for a six-mile run when it's ten below zero, my internal body temperature remains set—within a degree or two—at a fairly constant 98.6°F.

With hyperthermia treatment for cancer, a medication is first given to the patient to temporarily knock out the functioning of the thermoregulation center. The patient is then placed or submerged in a chamber or bath that heats up his or her body temperature to as high as 113°F for up to forty-five minutes.

Lo and behold, cancer cells get destroyed.[25]

With hyperthermia being a successful treatment for humans, especially in Europe—and with successful cases such as Ginger the boxer—I would hope hyperthermia is on the horizon for the future of companion animal cancer therapy. Targeted hyperthermia units are already available, though quite expensive, for treating cancer and other deep, chronic illnesses in animals.

Hyperthermia is often combined with other therapies such as radiation because, according to the National Cancer Institute, it "may make some cancer cells more sensitive to radiation or harm other cancer cells that radiation cannot damage. . . . Hyperthermia can also enhance the effects of certain anticancer drugs."[26]

In humans, hyperthermia therapy has been studied for the treatment of sarcoma, melanoma, and cancers of the head, neck, brain, lung, breast, liver, and many others. Tumor size has been significantly reduced by hyperthermia treatments—especially in conjunction with other therapies.

OXYGEN THERAPY

Simply stated, disease—especially cancer—either grows in and/or creates an oxygen-depleted environment. Therefore, supplying oxygen is a successful treatment for cancer and other disease states—both chronic and acute. When you think about it, this makes perfect sense. It's well-known that exercise and health go hand in hand. The main reason for this is that, during exercise, we breathe much higher levels of oxygen into our bodies. That's why it's called *aerobics*. Oxygen can be supplied through the following therapies:

Ozone therapy

One method of oxygenating cancer patients is through the use of the gas ozone, which is a molecule of oxygen with three oxygen atoms—O_3 (the oxygen molecule we breathe in the earth's atmosphere has two oxygen atoms, O_2). I wrote about ozone therapy in my first book, but I feel it is important enough to pass it along again.

Ozone can be administered via a number of different routes, including intravenously, by rectal catheter, by direct injection into a tumor, by injections into the abdominal cavity (called intraperitoneal), by filling a special bag that surrounds the patient from the head down, and by olive-oil salve that has been infused with high concentrations of the gas. One should seek consultation with an integrative veterinarian well experienced with this modality.

Food-grade hydrogen peroxide

Another way to administer oxygen therapy is through the use of what's known as food-grade hydrogen peroxide. Water is H_2O, while hydrogen peroxide adds another oxygen radical to become H_2O_2. The typical hydrogen peroxide you buy in a pharmacy is 3 percent strength, while food grade goes up to 35 percent hydrogen peroxide. This form of oxygen needs to be used with great caution because just a little of it can burn a hole in your hand. It can safely be taken through proper administration in drinking water, and some well-experienced practitioners administer it intravenously.

Hyperbaric oxygen therapy

One more approach to oxygen therapy is hyperbaric oxygen therapy—the patient breathes pure oxygen under pressure, most often in an enclosure called a hyperbaric chamber, or via a breathing tube. When oxygen is administered in a hyperbaric chamber, the pressure is three times higher (3 atm) than standard atmospheric pressure. This pushes more oxygen into the bloodstream—getting more oxygen into damaged tissues and cells and enhancing healing.

The use of hyperbaric oxygen therapy in dogs and cats mirrors for the most part its use in humans. This includes use in the following conditions—for some of which evidence of efficacy is strong, and for some in which use is still experimental:

- Anemia
- Crushing injury
- Nonhealing wounds
- Burns
- Gangrene
- Arthritis
- Decompression sickness
- Carbon monoxide poisoning
- Infection of skin or bone that causes tissue death

- Spinal cord injury
- Brain injury
- Cancer
- Radiation injury
- Allergies
- Heart disease
- Stroke

SPAY-NEUTER

Although this is not a New Age, alternative therapy, it's now scientifically proven that the right decision on *when* to spay can be more therapeutic than you might think. A spay-neuter is routinely done to most domesticated dogs and cats and is widely considered to be totally harmless. The truth turns out to be something different.

Doing this procedure at an early age, such as the typical six months, has been linked to major health issues, including adverse behavior and a number of chronic diseases. These diseases include a variety of orthopedic problems and increasing rates of certain cancer types. At one time, university studies claimed that we can and should be spaying and neutering as early as six to eight weeks of age. How horrible to stress animals that young and remove their sex hormones, which are so important to their development. We adopted one of our great cats, Topi, from a pet store. We tend to not do that, but it was love at first sight when we saw him. He was castrated at six weeks of age!

I once invited Dr. Christine Zink to guest on my Sirius

radio show. Dr. Zink is a Canadian-trained veterinarian who is a professor and director of the Department of Molecular and Comparative Pathobiology at the Johns Hopkins School of Medicine. Her specialty with dogs is orthopedic and sports medicine, and she has also conducted a number of studies related to the downsides of early spay and neuter. I could easily have spent half the show just reading her bio, which was twenty-seven typewritten pages long. What she shared about the tie of early spay-neuter to many of the common, but serious conditions veterinarians routinely encounter was eye-opening.

As a follow-up to this, the veterinary school at UC Davis published a comprehensive study conducted on 759 golden retrievers that has gained formidable acceptance across the veterinary profession.[27] The study basically advises against spaying and neutering dogs before one year of age. Although the outcome of the study is controversial, as with so many other issues like this, I lean toward avoiding spaying or neutering early in life. I believe this should apply to our feline friends, too.

ONE LAST THOUGHT ON HEALING PRACTICES

When I first started my acupuncture studies with the IVAS, two men made quite an impression on me and my concept of "being a healer." The first was a Dr. McKinnon from Canada, who shared with me his experience of studying in China. One small thing he said has stuck with me my entire career—especially when I started teaching others. He said that in China you don't learn by being lectured to. In China, you learn through a process of assimilation by observation!

The other gentleman, John Ottaviano, was rather young, but he had a remarkable amount of knowledge and experience in acupuncture. I recently learned that he has, unfortunately, passed. John and I became fast friends and dinner and drinking buddies. One night at dinner, I asked him how the heck he gained all this knowledge—especially at such a young age compared to the other lecturers. He told me that when he was in his midteens, he and two of his buddies were looking for a vocation and they stumbled upon an acupuncture master in San Francisco. The master told them if they wanted to learn, they would need to move into his house and serve him.

And that they did.

And that's *all* they did. Wash the toilets, clean the showers, make the meals—chore after chore. After several weeks, John's two friends dropped out from frustration, but he hung in there and just took care of the dirty work—week after week, wondering what the heck he had gotten himself into. Finally, after several months, the master said it was time. With the connection established between the two of them, the master transferred all his knowledge to John. And John got it.

Every time I think of this story, my mind immediately goes to the film *The Karate Kid* and the iconic "wax on, wax off" scene. I'm reminded that a tremendous amount of healing power can be found much deeper down than just on the physical plane where most of the effort to learn still exists.

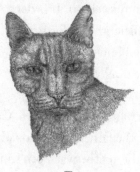

7

THE CURRENT STATE OF DOG AND CAT DISEASE

The physician should not treat the disease,
but the patient who is suffering from it.
—MOSES MAIMONIDES

What is disease and does it have a purpose?

We can begin to find an answer to those questions by first considering its derivation: "*dis*ease"—an uneasiness about the body.

And what is *-itis*?

-Itis is Latin for *inflammation*. You'll notice how many diseases end with *-itis*—hepatitis, arthritis, vasculitis, encephalitis, conjunctivitis, otitis, and on and on. There's a reason for that. The body creates inflammation as a part of healing and also detoxification, and we may not necessarily want to suppress these processes with drugs or other chemicals. If you get punched in the eye, twist your elbow, or cut

yourself, it's going to swell up. If it doesn't swell up, it's not going to heal as efficiently. Unfortunately, as a medical society, we have learned how to repress that -*itis*, and as a result we suppress the healing.

In my first book, I discuss Hering's Law of Cure. It's so important, it's worth mentioning again. Constantine Hering is considered to be the father of homeopathic medicine in the United States. Although he was born in Germany in 1800, he emigrated to Pennsylvania in 1833—starting a practice there and eventually founding the first school of homeopathy in the United States. According to Hering's Law of Cure, "All cure starts from within out, from the head down and in reverse order as the symptoms have appeared or been suppressed."[1] To get well, explains Hering, the patient must go through the crisis—expect it, look forward to it, and work toward it.

While there is no bible of natural healing principles—no Ten Commandments brought down from Mount Sinai by Moses—you might recall that I provided sixteen New Principles in the Spirit of Healing in chapter 1. Here are several that I think are worth highlighting in this chapter on disease:

- Before disease, there was health.
- Disease is not something that just happens to you or your animal companions, but something that you allow to happen, either consciously or unconsciously.
- An illness is nature's way of creating the fundamental conditions necessary for healing called homeostasis.
- Everything necessary for healing is built into every living

being. It's up to us to remove the obstacles to healing instead of adding new ones.

- Cancer is a confusion of nature caused mostly by man to now, in too many cases, outsmart himself.
- The immune system functions at its best when it is in a completely unaltered state.

We don't necessarily have to artificially stimulate an immune system (as with vaccines) because one of the primary laws of physics is that every action has an equal and opposite reaction. So, according to this law, by artificially stimulating one part of the immune system, another part of the immune system has to decline or even fail.

Here's a slightly revised and shortened version of one of the eighteen principles from my first book:

- Nature uses disease to reestablish a balance. Only when our bodies are out of balance are we subject to disease.

Homeostasis is the ability of an organism or cell to maintain internal equilibrium by adjusting its physiological processes. When the body is trying to reestablish homeostasis, it creates signs or symptoms of illness or disease.

In the sections that follow, I address some of the most significant diseases that I have encountered in my practice over the years. This is not meant to be an exhaustive list of every disease your dog or cat may encounter over his or her life. You can find that in my first book, or by consulting the internet, or especially in conjunction with your veterinarian. My intent here is to do a deep dive on several diseases that are particularly common and widespread—I want you to better understand them.

I owe much of my own education outside of veterinary school to a chiropractor I met way back in the seventies: Dr. George Zabrecky (he is now an MD and associate professor at the Sidney Kimmel Medical College at Thomas Jefferson University). He is by far the most brilliant person I have ever met in the practice of alternative medicine in conjunction with conventional medicine. His ability and knowledge are extraordinary. When he was a local, I would take my newly minted associated doctors out to dinner with Dr. Zabrecky, and they would pepper him with questions. He knew every answer and every possible aspect associated with that answer. He knew who won the Nobel Prize, what year the person won the Nobel Prize, the metabolic pathways involved with that Nobel Prize winner's research, every supplement that would modulate those pathways, and on and on. It's beyond comprehension what he knows.

Dr. Zabrecky has garnered the support of many advocates—most notable among them, Bernie Marcus, co-founder of The Home Depot. Following decades of Bernie's personal experiences with Dr. Zabrecky's integrative medical approaches, the Marcus Foundation decided to put significant support behind Dr. Zabrecky's research—culminating in the first Department of Integrative Medicine and Nutritional Sciences, located in the Sidney Kimmel Medical College at Thomas Jefferson University in Philadelphia.

HOMEOSTASIS

BY DR. GEORGE P. ZABRECKY

My initial memory regarding Dr. Martin Goldstein (Dr. Marty) was through patients who saw me for their health concerns and took their pets to Dr. Marty for similar alternative and integrative interventions. Although it was uncommon for physicians to practice nutritional care, it was rarer still in the veterinary arts. We are not just talking about providing a thoughtful diet of wholesome foods to support a pet's health; Dr. Marty could often make major, positive changes in the diseased animal population by the rational use of supplementation.

We have remained steadfast friends and colleagues from our initial meeting until the present (just over forty years). What I believe has connected Dr. Marty and me is our unwavering belief in homeostasis as a medical core concept.

This extraordinary property of the body has intrigued many physiologists. In 1865, Claude Bernard explained in his *Introduction to Experimental Medicine* that the "constancy of the internal milieu was the essential condition to a free life." But it was necessary to find a concept to link together the mechanisms that affected the regulation of the body. The credit for this concept goes to the American physiologist Walter Cannon. In 1932, impressed by "the wisdom of the body" capable of guaranteeing with such efficiency the control of the physiological equilibrium, Cannon coined the word *homeostasis* from two

Greek words meaning "to remain the same." Since then, the concept of homeostasis has had a central position in the field of medicine.

Homeostasis is one of the most remarkable and most typical properties of highly complex living organisms. A homeostatic system (an industrial firm, a large organization, a cell) is an open system that maintains its structure and functions by means of a multiplicity of dynamic equilibriums, rigorously controlled by interdependent regulation mechanisms. Such a system reacts to every change in the environment, or to every random disturbance, through a series of modifications of equal size and opposite direction to those that created the disturbance. The goal of these modifications is to maintain the internal balances.

Ecological, biological, and social systems are homeostatic. They oppose change with every means at their disposal. If the system does not succeed in reestablishing its equilibriums, it enters into another mode of behavior, one with constraints often more severe than the previous ones. This mode can lead to the destruction of the system if the disturbances persist.

Complex systems must have homeostasis to maintain stability and to survive. When injury or disease develops, the application of nutrients, through dietary modifications and supplementation, has enhanced the quality of life and longevity in all those that Dr. Marty has served.

THE C WORD

When I graduated Cornell in 1973, approximately 1 out of 10 dogs got cancer—it was always a disease of the old. If a young dog had a lump, we were taught to eliminate the possibility of cancer based solely on age. Today, the statistic is approximately 1 out of every 1.61 dogs in the United States will get some form of cancer, and not just older dogs.

This is particularly tragic when you consider the important role dogs and cats play in the lives of most people. As I mentioned earlier, Americans share their homes with some 90 million dogs and 94 million cats.[2] According to the 2019–20 APPA National Pet Owners Survey, 67 percent of US households have a pet. This works out to a total of 84.9 million homes with a pet—mostly a dog or a cat.[3]

As we'll discuss in chapter 9, dogs and cats possess a unique dynamic with the human race—one of unconditional love. However, we took the dynamic of the human race governed by unconditional love and turned it into cancer by creating an environment and approach that is toxic—both to us and to our animal companions. Just think!

Check out the below graph created by Dr. Carol Beuchat, founder of the Institute of Canine Biology. The graph charts the cancer rate in a variety of different mammals versus body mass—with special attention given to many dog breeds (marked with lighter gray dots). Particularly note the low incidence of cancer in other mammals such as elephants, tigers, and tree shrews, and the high incidence of cancer in many common dog breeds. One of these reasons is *domestication* and all that comes with that.

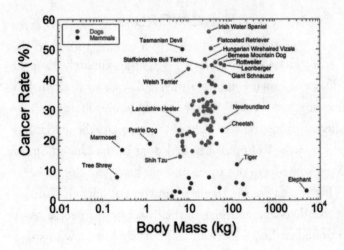

As Dr. Beuchat points out:

> Cancer is a problem not just in a few dog breeds but in many. Cancer rates of 20 percent or 30 percent are taken as "normal" because they are so much lower than the levels in breeds that are notorious for cancer—the ones up at 50 percent and 60 percent. Clearly, however, what is considered normal for dogs is much higher than what we see in mammals in general, and cancer rates that are "abnormally high" in dogs are actually off the charts.[4]

The Morris Animal Foundation—one of the most prominent animal research organizations in the profession of veterinary medicine, for which actress Betty White once served as president—has embarked on the Golden Retriever Lifetime Study with the aim of identifying nutritional, genetic, and environmental risk factors for cancer and other important diseases among our canine companions. More than three thousand golden retrievers are a part of the study, and the results thus far are quite interesting. In the 1970s, golden retrievers routinely lived up to sixteen or seventeen years. Today, that number has been whittled down to just nine or ten. A report published by the Golden Retriever Club of America says approximately 60 percent of all golden retrievers will die from cancer, and it's up to 66 percent for male goldens.[5]

My companion golden retriever, Daniel, lived to the ripe old age of nineteen. It's my deep hope that someday every golden—every dog and cat—will live this long or longer disease-free.

So what exactly is cancer? As we briefly touched on in chapter 1, simplistically stated, cancer is a lack of proper cell differentiation. During the earliest stage of development in mammals—humans, cats, dogs—the cells are all the same. These are the stem cells we hear so much about. They have the potential to become any sort of cell in the body. However, all of a sudden, nature flips a switch and these stem cells begin to *differentiate*—that is, they specialize to become muscle cells, intestinal cells, eyeballs, heart, brain. It's a miracle of nature, and certainly something that man—with all his technological advances—can't come close to doing, except maybe in Hollywood.

Think about it. Because of an immunological foul-up, cells trying to form normal new bone grow in an aberrated, uncontrolled manner. They resemble bone but are wildly distorted and lack normal structure and function, and they unfortunately have the ability to uncontrollably grow and kill. As a result, when we're looking for what causes cancer, we shouldn't be focusing on the tumor, but instead on the things that foul up the immune system so the body can't properly complete cell differentiation. So, what are these factors that screw things up and suppress the immune system?

In my forty-five years of veterinary experience, I have found three significant influences on that:

1. **Vaccinations.** I am not anti-vaccination, but the vaccination protocols we've established in veterinary medicine have become immune suppressive. Calling dogs and cats into veterinary offices every three years—or even every single year—for all their vaccines, and with no dose-to-weight relationship for vaccines, just doesn't make sense. Why is a 2-pound Chihuahua given the exact same dose as a 140-pound Great Dane? By the way, it's been scientifically proven that the dose that the Great Dane gets could be up to ten times what it needs. We'll dig deeper into vaccinations in the next chapter.

2. **Diet.** Certain diets supply the energy that grows cancer cells. In chapter 4, we explored proper diet in great detail. If you feed your animal companions quality food that's biologically appropriate and avoid feeding them glyphosates and GMOs and other unnatural substances, then you'll be giving them the tools they need to allow Mother Nature to keep them healthy and happy. Dr. Gregory Ogilvie is a leading veterinary oncologist who proved scientifically that certain by-products of grain or cereal metabolism in the sugar family support the growth of cancer cells in the dog's body.[6] As you'll recall, the standard dog kibble is usually high in grain and cereal, especially corn.

3. **Genetics.** While you can't do anything about genetics within one lifetime, we humans have not done our animal companions any favors here. We've degraded the earth, spewed toxins into the air, land, and water—creating a constant assault on the DNA of every organism on this planet, including ourselves. In addition, we've made so many mistakes in health care for so many decades that we commonly see young dogs—even as young as three months of age—with serious cancer. They're either born with a tumor or with a genetic predisposition to rapidly form cancer. In the majority of cases, I believe it's the latter and not the former.

Ultimately, cancer is an aberration of nature caused by man—it is *not* a natural condition. I love dinosaurs, and I thought of becoming a paleontologist before choosing to become a veterinarian. It's therefore no big surprise that I am also a big fan of Michael Crichton, the author of *Jurassic Park*. He earned his MD at Harvard and had a unique understanding of science and medicine that made his books much more credible than the work of most other authors in the genre. Sadly, Crichton was diagnosed with lymphoma in early 2008, and the cancer killed him within about six months.

In *Jurassic Park*, Crichton introduces chaos theory to readers, mapping a series of iterations that explain why what happened at the amusement park happened.

First iteration: "At the earliest drawings of the fractal curve, few clues to the underlying mathematical structure will be seen." —Ian Malcolm

Second iteration: "With subsequent drawings of the fractal curve, sudden changes may appear." —Ian Malcolm

Third iteration: "Details emerge more clearly as the fractal curve is redrawn." —Ian Malcolm

Fourth iteration: "Inevitably, underlying instabilities begin to appear." —Ian Malcolm

Fifth iteration: "Flaws in the system will now become severe." —Ian Malcolm

Sixth iteration: "System recovery may prove impossible." —Ian Malcolm

Seventh iteration: "Increasingly, the mathematics will demand the courage to face its implications." —Ian Malcolm

Michael Crichton's point was simple: Bringing back creatures into modern times that lived on this planet hundreds of millions of years ago was such an unnatural act that it *had* to fail. The failure wasn't just because of the guy (Newman from *Seinfeld*) who left the gate unlatched in the rainstorm— leading to the escape of the reconstituted dinosaurs. If it weren't that, something else would have failed.

The same holds true with cancer. If you mess so much with nature, with all the things we described—the vaccines, improper diet, chemical suppression by drugs, environmental pollution, and much more—this unnatural disease called cancer *had* to happen, just like the dinosaurs in *Jurassic Park*. Cancer actually is the sixth and seventh iterations, where system (the immune system) recovery may prove impossible, and the mathematics demand courage to face its implications. I believe the idea applies to diseases such as AIDS, SARS, and the recent COVID-19 pandemic.

One of the key tenets of cancer treatment is that early detection and removal give you a better chance of recovery. This, of course, is not entirely correct. If it was, then every animal with cancer that was detected early and removed would survive to a ripe, old age. We know that's not the case at all. Another key tenet of cancer treatment is that the surgeon should try to get as wide a margin around the cancer as he or she can. The fallacy of wide margins is finally getting traction in conventional medicine, and this is something I've been promoting for many years. Before an individual gets cancer, they *are* a wide margin.

Where did the first cancer cell come from? The garage? The Bronx?

No. The first cancer cell came from a normal cell that started to go crazy. We all have the potential.

So, the more you try to cure cancer by removing or zapping it, the farther away you're going from the causative effect of cancer.

What, then, is the cure for cancer?

It's not in a laboratory.

It's not in a test tube.

It's *definitely* not in a drug company.

It doesn't cost trillions of dollars a year.

It does exist.

It's called . . .

HEALTH!

When I walk through this thought process in a talk, I'll often say how many times I've heard, "Boy, if it wasn't for his tumor, he was in great shape!" To me, cancer is the ultimate level of a lack of health. So again, instead of working to treat the cancer, look to maintain health. An individual who is healthy—be it animal or human—*does not* have cancer.

So, with this in mind, how do we care for a cancer patient?

If your animal companion is unfortunately diagnosed with this horrible disease, the first thing you need to do is not become the target of the "C-word." Doing so puts you in the position of passively becoming just an *effect* while cancer goes into the driver's seat as *cause*. *Cancer* has become such a horrible word in the foundation of our society—one that imparts a tremendous amount of gut-wrenching fear and loathing—that I propose we just change the word. Rational thought is not as common when you function in the lower emotional bands of fear, despair, and denial.

Proper care for a cancer patient begins with establishing a sense of hope. In dealing with many thousands of cancer patients over my career, the first thing I do is build hope in these understandably distraught pet parents. I introduce them to some of my most remarkable before-and-after cases, some truly astounding, so they can take the hopelessness they feel (often sparked by less optimistic veterinarians and even oncologists) and displace it with a feeling that something *can* be done. And I am not talking about false hope. We need to be "real" when properly dealing with this disease. As I said before, doing just this alone has caused a small level of improvement in many patients I have seen over my career. This will be more evident when you read Elsa's story at the end of this chapter.

The next step is to consult with a veterinarian who is well experienced in dealing with cancer patients, possibly even an oncologist if indicated. Please do not attempt to treat your cancer patient with Dr. Google or by utilizing other internet sources. Sure, research to your heart's content, but also go one step further and consult with a real veterinarian who is skilled in the treatment of cancer. Believe me, if I was ever diagnosed with cancer, I would not attempt to treat myself with online resources!

One of the first things I will typically ask a cancer patient's parent is "What is the most predictable thing about cancer, patient to patient?" Typically, the answer I get is "My dog is going to die" or "The tumor will continue to grow and grow and grow."

Nope! Those are not the correct answers.

I will then show them case reports of pets given months to live by some of the top oncologists in the country who now live happy and good lives four, six, even more than nine years later. That would be similar to a human diagnosed with terminal cancer living another fifty years.

So, the correct answer to my question is "The most predictable thing about cancer, patient to patient, is that it is almost totally unpredictable." Yes, some statistics provide estimates. But predictability? Nope.

I have had several patients of about the same age who were diagnosed with the exact same cancer. One will live just three months, while another will live four or five years or more. Why? I believe that cancer is a man-made, or at minimum a man-influenced, condition. In most cases, the innate intelligence of cancer now exceeds that of the humans who created or influenced it. It does whatever the hell it wants to do whenever it wants, despite the formerly powerful immune systems contained within us and our animal companions, and despite the trillions of dollars spent to try to stop it. And unfortunately for us, it does not observe weekends and holidays. Take it from me—it's been my life for forty-five years.

What about conventional modalities of cancer treatment? Keep in mind that we are or should be deeply set in the wonderful world of integrative medicine. As much as I am in favor of alternative, less invasive therapies, I have seen thousands of lives saved conventionally. What I'm not in favor of is holistic veterinarians who jump on the bandwagon just because they're recommending a couple of supplements, inappropriately stopping needed conventional therapy, and improperly treating patients. It's these veterinarians that I call "assholistic."

Conventional treatments can in many cases be useful for buying the time we need to work on the real cause of the tumor's growth—the immune system. If a tumor is blocking a vital function of life and can be removed surgically or zapped by radiation to save the patient's life, then by all means do it. This is where it is vital to work hand in hand with a well-experienced integrative veterinarian to receive this proper guidance.

Cancer and fear certainly go hand in hand. I have had thousands of pet parents allow fear to stop them from doing a surgery that's necessary for their pet's long-term survival. "But what if she doesn't make it through the procedure?" they'll ask me. The answer is that, without taking a leap of faith, she simply has no chance to live much longer. Please, let's look at her glass as half full, not half empty.

Conventional chemotherapy and radiation work by creating high levels of free radicals to destroy the cancer. Antioxidants are free-radical scavengers. In scientific theory, it's an absolute no-no to give antioxidants to a cancer patient undergoing conventional chemotherapy or radiation. However, many years ago my friend George Zabrecky gave me a packet of papers with well over a hundred references for how cancer patients undergoing conventional therapy do better while taking antioxidants. This research is becoming more widely accepted by conventional veterinarians.

The way I see it, chemotherapy and radiation are so strong in their effect that not many things are going to get in the way of creating enough free radicals to destroy the cancer. These free radicals also gain access to the rest of the body, so the patient suffers. Why are there so many side effects with chemotherapy and radiation? Because the free radicals aren't just staying in the tumor. So, by administering antioxidants, you're tremendously supporting the patients while they undergo chemotherapy and radiation.

When I'm working with an oncologist—and when I'm treating a cancer patient who is also being treated by an oncologist—I usually put the oncologist and his or her therapy in the driver's seat. I then take the back seat to support the patient during the therapy. Not only does this help the patient, but it helps smooth relationships governed by ego. I also share with the client that, even though it's sacrilegious in oncology to use antioxidants on a patient undergoing chemotherapy and radiation treatments, tons of scientific evidence now shows that patients undergoing these therapies have a better success rate using antioxidants. I suggest that my clients share this knowledge with their oncologist.

Remember, there are more ways than just one magic bullet to treat any diseased patient. What works for one may not work for another, so you must always have an open mind and be ready to try different approaches and shift gears quickly.

One of the nicknames I have given to cancer, even in the successful patient, is "roller coaster." Cancer is not reversed overnight, but by life and the slow reestablishment of the integrity of the immune system to again properly care for itself on a cellular level. As the body and immune system strengthen, the immune system can then turn toward a deeper level of disease and toxicity. Just as Hering set forth ages ago, healing will itself create disease. He didn't call it a healing "crisis" for nothing!

Since our animal companions are direct reflections of our emotional states, it is vital to learn how to ride this roller coaster rather than have it ride you. Again, do your best to stay in the driver's seat of cause and not the back seat of effect.

Another nickname I give cancer is "relativity." How a cancer patient is doing is so often a relative thing. Subtle reminders of this along the way can be a huge benefit to the emotional state of the pet parent that we just learned is also so critical. Many times a dog has come to me previously diagnosed by another veterinarian or oncologist as having a serious cancer and given just weeks or a few months to live. When three years later that dog is still alive—mostly enjoying life, but still with the tumor—and Mom or Dad asks, "Do you think it's working?," my answer is an unequivocal *yes!* That's why I wrote the second New Principle in the Spirit of Healing: "With any degenerative condition, stability in the face of expected decline is actually improvement."

Also, along these lines, so many parents of ill patients

have asked me, as we start a program, "What should I look for?" Although many symptoms can manifest along the way, I have made it a firm habit to never give people negative things to look for. The mind is a powerful thing, as is the human-animal bond. So, I almost always say, "Look for how great she is doing!"

When an animal gets ill in its natural state, the typical recourse is for it to quickly go off on its own and find a protected place to partially hibernate. When people have a bad cold or flu, do they typically go to the hospital or to bed? And what happens to their appetite when they get sick? It is suppressed. How unfortunate it is that we do not grant millions of companion animals this same right.

I am not saying do not bring your sick companion animal to your veterinarian for proper diagnosis and treatment. I just want to reiterate that disease—a fever, a discharge, even an ache—has a purpose. And as in the example of a person with a cold, not all illnesses need to be diagnosed and treated, especially with medications that stop nature's curative processes and themselves have side effects. This is a tough call, even for me with over forty-five years of experience. That is why working with a veterinarian trained in integrative medicine is a huge help.

One of the most unfortunate things about cancer is that it is a confusion of nature, created by man. A diabetic has high blood sugar because of a lack of insulin. The diabetic's cells are starving for proper levels of glucose to function because insulin is required to transport glucose from the bloodstream to the cells. We have a similar effect with cancer. Since the immune system is composed of proteins called immunoglobulins, it becomes starved for protein. And where does it go looking for protein? The muscles. That is why cancer is a wasting or emaciating disease. Just think what a person who has just passed away due to cancer looks like. Gaunt. Thin. A shadow of their former selves. And because the patient is ill, their natural tendency is to fast.

So as much as I like to feed cancer patients the healthy diet we discussed in chapter 4—high-quality meat protein, some veggies, and little to no cereal products—a rule of thumb for feeding a cancer patient who is anorectic is "any food is better than no food." You want and need to break this cycle of anorexia.

Now the fun begins: setting a course for proper therapy. Start by reestablishing proper life function if needed. If the only way to do this is surgery, chemotherapy, or radiation—because without it the patient will continue to suffer or die—then by all means choose one of those therapies. One of the most important aspects of any successful patient is *time*. So what if it takes years to successfully treat a cancer patient? As long as the quality of life is worth living, then that's fine!

When people come to me after being told their animal companion doesn't have long to live, and I go over the comprehensive, labor-intensive program that they will need to administer, I'm often asked, "How long do we have to do this?"

My response is usually something like "Maybe five more years."

At first, they grimace after hearing those words. But once it sinks in and they get it, and they start to beam, I respond, "Yeah, won't that be great!"

THE CURRENT STATE OF DOG AND CAT DISEASE · 203

Again, bringing in a bit of levity when dealing with the scourge of cancer can only help to lift everyone's spirits. I have *no* affinity for being serious. I am not saying that conditions such as cancer or global pandemics should, at all, be taken lightly. It's just that outcomes are not as promising when they are confronted with the emotional solidness of being serious. I feel that so many problems on this planet stem from the terminal condition called "seriousness."

Over my career, the strongest and most effective alternative way I've found to go at the cancer itself—but also to not set the patient back—is the intravenous vitamin C therapy discussed in chapter 6. Even though it does have beneficial effects just days or months later, it alone is not a "cure" for cancer.

I wrote a section in my first book about cryosurgery—the controlled freezing of cancer cells/tumors. With the wonders I have experienced observing and using cryosurgery over my entire career—since the early days when I watched my brother, Bob, develop it as a modality for our profession, to its use today—I don't understand why it has not caught on in veterinary medicine to the extent it should have. In a nutshell, cryosurgery has some significant advantages over conventional surgery, when applicable. Typically, cryosurgery

- Is less invasive
- Results in less bleeding
- Requires less sedation or anesthesia
- Is tissue sparing
- Is the only form of surgery that has an immune-stimulating

effect, both locally when the tissue is frozen and more systemically throughout the immune system

- Can successfully get to and destroy a tumor from within where conventional surgery cannot because there are no borders to cut *around* it to effectively remove

There are now tons of nutraceuticals with claims to be anticancer and/or immune supportive. We've explored in this book some of my personal favorites, including artemisinin, medicinal mushrooms, CBD products, and others. In addition, in my first book I explored Poly-MVA and others. But there are a multitude, and this is where working hand in hand with an experienced integrative veterinarian comes into play. I truly do not want to limit this book by listing just my several favorites when not only are there so many today, but over time—way after this book is published—many more will be discovered or created. Plus, I guarantee that there are many of which I am either not aware or have no experience using.

And remember the company MediVet, from chapter 6? The company offers a promising service for the treatment of cancer in dogs: K9-ACV or canine autologous cancer vaccine. The veterinarian takes cells from a patient's malignant tumor and sends them to MediVet. Then MediVet creates a personalized vaccine from it—stimulating the dog's own immune system to attack that specific cancer. According to MediVet, the treatment is both safe and clinically effective.

I consider one book to be my bible for treating cancer: *The Dog Cancer Survival Guide,* coauthored by two of my dear colleagues, Dr. Demian Dressler and board-certified oncologist Dr. Sue Ettinger. Besides containing a wealth of information on specifically treating cancer patients, this book is a must for any pet lover's library shelf. And within this book you will learn about another of my favorite anticancer supplements, Apocaps, which was created by Dr. Dressler. This supplement—which contains botanical extracts and other natural ingredients—is specifically formulated to support apoptosis, the natural process by which the body eliminates spent cells from itself.

As Dr. Ian Billinghurst so wisely points out, a lot of the treatment options for cancer focus only on the cancer. The doctors want to kill the cancer, but they forget that the cancer lives in a dog, cat, or other companion animal. We veterinarians are a disease-oriented profession. However, I know that I have not forgotten that cancer lives in a dog or a cat, and my own focus—and the focus of every good veterinarian—is squarely on the health and well-being of our patients.

During a webinar for *Dogs Naturally Magazine,* I was reminded about a presentation I gave with my friend and colleague Rodney Habib (more about him in chapter 10). I explained in my presentation that, when dealing with cancer that is manifest in the body, we should always keep the focus on the patient and life—both in dogs that have cancer and those that do not—and not allow the focus to be pulled toward cancer and death.

When I prescribe Poly-MVA or artemisinin for a patient, clients will often ask, "Do you take this yourself—or give it to your dogs—to prevent cancer?" I say, "No, in a healthy patient, I never do *anything* in reference to cancer. I take things to stay healthy. I don't allow cancer to exist in any form in myself or in my patients' universe—physically, or somewhere in the extraphysical plane mentally, emotionally, and especially spiritually. I only focus on health." Therefore, I wouldn't take an anticancer supplement to prevent cancer because, if I did, then I just created a place in the universe for cancer to exist. Don't focus on the darkness, but instead bring the light.

I remember listening years ago to a well-versed integrative doctor who was being interviewed on a SiriusXM radio show. The interviewer asked, "What would you do if you were diagnosed with cancer?" The doctor said, "I wouldn't call my doctor; I'd call my travel agent."

Unfortunately, I have to agree with him. If I were ever to get cancer, my first consideration would be to leave the country. Germany and Switzerland have some of the more successful doctors who treat these severe illnesses. I visited the Paracelsus Clinic in Switzerland, and what they do there in the field of advanced alternative therapies made a lasting imprint on me. I also spent four days at the Sanoviv Medical Institute in Mexico, where I was invited to speak. While there, I immersed myself in their health program and felt better than I had in years.

At our clinic, we have animals that came to us five, six, seven years ago with, for example, tumors in their abdomen and prognoses of just a few months to live. Most were transformed into happy and active survivors. The cancer didn't kill them, but they still have tumors in their abdomen—we can feel or sonogram them. So, we've been unsuccessful in reference to the cancer—we didn't eradicate it. However, we've been very successful in reference to the patient. These dogs and cats are acting healthy, aside from the tumor they've been carrying with them for many years.

Here's another thing about a cancer patient who has a tumor. As we discussed, it is easy to go at the effect of that tumor on your animal companion, and the quicker it's gone, the better you will feel. Many times, depending on the individual case, if a tumor is present—and it can be easily monitored and is not highly aggressive nor negatively affecting the life or function of the patient—I like to leave it there.

Why? Two reasons.

First, as already discussed, we don't work so much on the cancer as we do on the patient and his/her immune system. Having the tumor there serves as a marker. If it's shrinking or at least stable, it's a great sign of what's going on systemically, and especially to what could be happening on the inside that can't easily be detected.

The second reason is even more important. When I discuss this with clients, I usually start by asking them, "What is the number one stimulus to the immune system in the body of a cancer patient?" Rarely does anyone answer this correctly. The correct answer is the tumor or cancerous process itself. I learned this so well from the genius I wrote about in my first book, Dr. Lawrence Burton. (Sadly, Dr. Burton passed away in 1993, and the Immune Augmentation Therapy, or IAT, program we tried to permanently establish in our clinic—and which I wrote about extensively in my first book—had to be shut down.) Dr. Burton scientifically proved that there is a tumor antibody system. Just as the number one stimulus to the immune system when an individual gets exposed to a virus or a bacterium is the invading organism itself, a tumor cell produces a protein that he termed *tumor complement*. This in turn stimulates the production by the immune system of an immunoglobulin.

This is why I believe the stories I've heard of people who have had a small tumor growing slowly on their arm or other body part over a few years, and they decide to have it removed. Just a few months later, you hear that the person died of systemic cancer. I believe that the tumor was stimulating the production of tumor antibodies—not only holding that tumor in check, but also preventing other cells in the body from becoming cancerous. When you suddenly remove the tumor and it no longer releases any tumor complement, all these other hidden cells start to proliferate immediately— overwhelming the immune system and the individual.

So, I usually recommend leaving the tumor there, working on the patient's immune system, and monitoring both closely. If it continues to grow despite those efforts, then by all means get it removed. And as I already explained, I am not a big fan of cancer-spread theory and the idea that the faster you get a tumor out, with wide margins, the better your chances of preventing spread and of effecting a cure. As I said, if cancer does in fact spread throughout the body from that tumor, where did the first cell spread from? The garage?

Remember: Where intention goes, energy flows. If you keep your head and your heart in the right frame of mind and spirit, you have a better chance to keep the doors closed to cancer and other terrible diseases—both in yourself and in your animal companions. As you will see in chapter 9, we share a strong bond with our dog and cat companions on both a physical and extraphysical level, one in which disease can be affected.

My good friend and colleague Dr. Ian Billinghurst—originator of the biologically appropriate raw food (BARF) diet we explored in chapter 4—is one of the world's leading experts on the origins of cancer. It's a complex topic, but I think you'll find Dr. Billinghurst's perspective to be both right on and interesting in its conclusions—especially his tracing of the origins of cancer back 2 billion years.

CANCER . . . ITS EVOLUTIONARY ORIGINS AND SOLUTION

BY DR. IAN BILLINGHURST

Four billion years ago (4 BYA), in a galaxy called the Milky Way, on the planet Earth, a single-celled creature called Luca appeared. Her default state was constant reproduction. And this became the default state for all future life on earth. Today, every cell in every organism has the constant urge to reproduce itself. This urge, for all differentiated cells, in mammals, such as dogs, cats, and humans, is kept under control by a bewildering array of checks and balances, brought about by billions of years of evolution.

Before Luca disappeared (around 3.7 BYA), she had produced two children: Bacteria and Archaea. Luca, Bacteria, and Archaea belonged to one tribe, the Prokaryotes, or primitive single-celled creatures. All three had the default state of constant reproduction. And they had another common trait. Unstable DNA. Without DNA repair mechanisms and because their DNA was not protected by a nuclear membrane, their DNA was constantly mutating.

Around 2 BYA, the Bacteria and Archaea gave birth to the Eukaryotes. The Eukaryote tribe (whose default state continued to be constant reproduction) gave rise to all multicellular forms of life, including dogs, cats, and humans. This was only possible because the bacterial ancestor had become a powerful energy-producing organelle, the mitochondrion. It produced energy (ATP) by burning proteins, fats, and sugars; a process called aerobic respiration.

Eukaryotes also produced ATP by fermentation (or glycolysis), a process that only burns sugar. When food was plentiful, Eukaryotes used fermentation to produce ATP. This spared the proteins and fats, making them available to be used as building blocks for the new cells. When food was scarce, Eukaryotes used aerobic respiration, burning all their food just to stay alive, and reproduction ceased. A genetic program linking ATP production to the reproductive state became embedded in the DNA of the Eukaryotes; it remains today in all mammals, only switched on when fermentation becomes a cell's principal way of producing ATP. For example, early embryonic stem cells—where ATP is produced by fermentation—express their default state of constant reproduction. Similarly, when a tissue stem cell is forced to produce its ATP by fermentation, the tissue we call cancer is initiated.

This process begins when carcinogens—and/or aberrant lifestyle—damage a tissue stem cell's unprotected mitochondrial DNA (not the highly protected nuclear DNA, as currently—and erroneously—believed). Where the resulting damage is acute, the cell dies for lack of energy and cancer is not initiated. Chronic damage occasionally results in survival via the up-regulation of fermentation. This initiates the cell's preexisting genetic program of reproduction, which includes the removal of DNA repair mechanisms. This stem cell has returned to its default state of ceaseless reproduction and mutations.

Because cancer arises following a stem cell's switch to producing its ATP by fermentation (initiating a preexisting genetic program of reproduction), it may be destroyed by starvation, using tools such as ketosis and calorie restriction. Given the universal applicability, availability, cheapness, effectiveness, and humanity of this approach . . . why do we ignore it?[7]

DENTAL DISEASE

With all that I've studied since the writing of my first book, this is such an important aspect of health that I feel it is worth reexploring. Yes, it's well-known that periodontal disease can have a negative impact on the health of your animal companion's heart, kidneys, and liver. But periodontal disease has also been found, especially in European studies, to have a negative impact on the immune system.

I have long been aware that some of the most successful doctors specializing in cancer therapy in Germany started therapy by removing their cancer patients' amalgam fillings and root-canal-filled teeth—and at times most if not all the teeth. Dr. Hans Nieper and Dr. Josef Issels were proponents of this approach. Once mercury fillings and root-canaled teeth were removed, the patients' immune functions appeared to improve significantly. According to Dr. Issels, during his forty-year practice of treating terminally ill cancer patients, 97 percent of the cancer patients in his care had root canals. Although this approach still sounds a bit extreme to me, it revealed the tie between chronic deep dental disease and immune suppression. This is why maintaining the dental health of your animal companions is vital to their overall health.

In addition, after attending continuing-education courses and wet labs in veterinary dentistry, I learned some important things that I didn't understand well earlier in my career. The instructors would show photographs of dogs with bad tartar, then they would show photos of the teeth cleaned spotlessly, then photographs of X-rays taken of these same dogs. We could see micro-abscesses, resorption of the roots, and a lot of disease. In the old days when we would see dogs with tartar, we'd chip it off and their teeth looked great. But we were never looking underneath.

I do need to correct what I wrote in my first book about chipping off tartar and bypassing the use of sedation. While this would be okay in a younger dog or cat with basically healthy teeth and gums and mild tartar, in most cases proper sedation, evaluation, and handling is vital. My only caveat to this is the reemergence of the Houndstooth method of non-anesthetic dental cleanings for dogs and cats (www.houndstoothpetdental.com). As I write this book, Houndstooth has locations in eight states with the hopes of going national.

Although not appropriate for all cases of dental disease, Houndstooth is a good way for maintaining ongoing dental health while avoiding sedation, especially in some older patients where general anesthesia could pose a health risk. Houndstooth's unique method gets deeper into the periodontal area under the gums than other methods. I have observed a number of procedures performed by veterinary technicians licensed in the Houndstooth method. Besides their skills at cleaning the teeth and under the gums in the periodontal zone with their instruments, the key is their method of gentle restraint, which allows them, on most of the animal cleanings I have witnessed, to perform this technique without sedation.

One other aspect of proper dental health became evident to me over the last two decades through personal experience. In my youth, I never knew much about proper dental health. I should have had braces, should not have kept my wisdom teeth until I was in my sixties, should have learned about flossing at a much younger age, and should not have thought as a kid that a triple-X hardness toothbrush—rubbed across my teeth as hard as I could, to the point of wearing away some enamel—was the way to go. That's when I turned to my own holistic dentist, Dr. David Lerner, to slowly help me correct so many of the mistakes I had made.

David is a master at reflexive kinesiology. As he worked with me, I was stunned how he would go over my body kinesiologically, determine weak reflexes, then pinpoint those to specific teeth in my mouth. He would then have me bite down on a cotton sponge on that tooth, and my reflex would strengthen tremendously. As a result, I started to grasp how the mouth is an energetic Grand Central Station for the rest of the body. I invited David to be a guest on one of my *Ask Martha's Vet* SiriusXM satellite-radio shows. He shared with the listening audience an experiment conducted in Japan in which dogs were intentionally made to have bite stress by the grinding down of their teeth. Within a short time, all of them developed joint problems and disease.

This is why I invited David to contribute the sidebar that follows.

THE DENTAL CONNECTION IN ANIMALS

BY DAVID L. LERNER, DDS

The Center for Holistic Dentistry[8]

Human beings and the animals we love have much in common. Research into the genetics of dogs and cats show that they are similar to us, sharing the vast majority of our genes. The similarities are so strong that we can also suffer many of the same diseases. The top ten diseases that affect us humans are also the top-ten diseases among purebred dogs, including cancer, heart disease, epilepsy, allergies, retinal disease, and cataracts.

While tooth decay is common in humans, it is uncommon in dogs and even less so in cats and other animals. This is because tooth decay is the result of acidic conditions in the mouth in response to diet—and the growth of specific bacterial strains that thrive on refined carbohydrates—that dissolve the hardened mineralized surface in enamel. The saliva of dogs and cats as well as horses is significantly more alkaline and therefore more protective against dental decay, and their diets generally should not include refined carbohydrates.

Gum disease is as common in domesticated animals as in humans, maybe more so, because their diets are so different from that of similar animals in the wild. It is estimated that 85 percent of dogs and cats over four years of age have periodontal disease. One-third of all horses have some gum disease, and over 60 percent of horses over thirteen years of age have severe periodontal disease.

Gum disease is caused by the invasion of bacteria into our gums causing inflammation and bone destruction. The biofilm that accumulates—called dental plaque—can change in character over time if not removed, favoring the growth of more invasive bacterial species.

Research by Weston Price, DDS, found that humans who ate a natural diet experienced many fewer gum issues than their counterparts who ate a processed diet. Francis Pottenger, MD, did a famous study that showed the decline in health of cats fed a cooked diet versus those fed a raw diet.

We now know that in humans, periodontal disease is a contributor to many chronic ailments due to the invasion of bacteria through blood vessels to the heart and brain, as well as the toxic effects of their waste products. This all contributes to chronic inflammation throughout the human body.

In humans, conditions such as heart disease and cancer of the colon, pancreas, and prostate have all been shown to have common links with periodontal disease. Diabetes and obesity, stroke, lung disease, kidney disease, the autoimmune diseases, and adverse outcomes of pregnancy have also been documented to have connections with periodontal disease. It seems reasonable, given the genetic similarities, that there would be similar consequences in animals as well.

What then are the consequences of tooth loss in our beloved animal companions? Loss of teeth will result in loss of support for the jaw muscles, with a potential for a chain of events that further contributes to the decline of the dog's or cat's health, just as we see in humans.

Equine veterinary medicine recognizes that it may be necessary to adjust the shape of a horse's teeth so they wear evenly and maintain balanced forces on the teeth and jaw muscles. Maintaining balance in the horse's bite is important to maintaining balance in the horse's gait.

Studies done with rats, guinea pigs, and dogs showed that loss of support of the back teeth resulted in a shifting of the bite. This in turn changed muscular balance and tone throughout the body, from head to tail. In addition, the functioning of the autonomic nervous system and endocrine system shifted, resulting in diminished vitality of all of the body's systems. The same is seen in humans.

Here's one last thing I would like to share. I attended the 2016 American Holistic Veterinary Medical Association's annual conference in Columbus, Ohio, with my dear friend Cindy Meehl and the entire film crew from *The Dog Doc* documentary to capture some key footage. While there, one of the lectures Cindy and I attended was given by a knowledgeable, certified veterinary dentist from San Diego, Dr. Brook Niemiec. Within the first few minutes of the lecture, he said words that blew me away and still remain music to my ears: "We no longer prescribe antibiotics for most of our patients."

I leaned over to Cindy and said, "What? Am I hearing this correctly?"

Dr. Niemiec explained that, during typical periodontal disease conditions, a biofilm is created, and this biofilm very strongly prevents the absorption of antibiotics into the area. The only way to get the antibiotics anywhere near the area of concern is to first break down this biofilm with proper scaling, typically with an ultrasonic device. However, once this is done, and the area becomes that much cleaner, the antibiotic treatment is not needed. Exceptions would depend on the severity of the infection's access to other parts of the body.

Today, this approach has become the accepted norm in veterinary dentistry—something I have been a proponent of for decades.

ALLERGIES

I believe that somewhere around 85 percent of all disease in humans is not only underlain by some sort of allergy or autoimmune condition, but that about an equal percentage of our companion animal population is plagued with similar medical conditions.

Most of us probably don't think much about the allergies we have until they hit us hard, such as during allergy season, when a lot of pollen is in the air. Then, all of a sudden, we're suffering from a runny nose, nasal congestion, itchy, watery eyes, sneezing, and more. An inconvenience, but no big deal—right? Wrong. According to the Asthma and Allergy Foundation of America, more than 50 million Americans deal with allergies every year, and allergies are the sixth leading cause of chronic illness in the United States—costing the nation more than $18 billion a year.[9]

In both humans and our animal companions, allergies are triggered when the body's immune system mistakenly identifies its own cells as foreign and then initiates an inflammatory reaction against them—often including the production of autoantibodies. We sensitize the body's cells to become allergic to a foreign protein such as pollen. Secondarily to that, we're sensitizing the body's own cells to attack other cells in the body—this is autoimmune disease. Allergies can take place in the gastrointestinal system, the joints, the skin, the respiratory system, or any other place in the body. Triggers can include a variety of things, including food, flea saliva, environmental allergens including dust, pollen, mold, trees, grasses, and much more.

But to gain a better understanding of allergies, I believe we need to look at what actually sensitizes the immune system to react to a specific element—especially some foreign protein, or even to its own cells—causing the inflammatory reaction we've come to call allergy. And, more specifically, what sensitizes a normal blood cell called the mast cell to release histamines, which actually cause allergy symptoms. While pollen may trigger a response in some people, others will be unaffected. (For decades, I have run through fields full of clouds of pollen and other allergens with no ill effect.) Why is that? Why are the bodies of some humans, dogs, and cats tricked into thinking their own cells are enemy organisms that must be destroyed?

On a broad level, one thing comes to mind: vaccinations. When I think of the term *autoimmune disease,* I feel that it is synonymous with the most prominent documented adverse reactions to vaccinations. A team at Purdue University College of Veterinary Medicine looked into whether vaccines can alter the immune systems of dogs—leading to life-threatening immune-mediated diseases. The vaccinated dogs in this study developed "significantly elevated concentrations" of autoantibodies to many of their own biochemicals, including fibronectin, laminin, DNA, albumin, cytochrome c, cardiolipin, and collagen. The nonvaccinated dogs did not.[10] In another study, puppies vaccinated for canine distemper before being given pollen extracts had many more immunoglobulin E (IgE) antibodies than did their control littermates who were not vaccinated until after the last pollen extract injection.[11] A medical term now categorizes this process: *allergic breakthrough phenomenon.*[12]

Just after I presented the manuscript for my first book to my publisher in 1999, I found a startling research paper (that unfortunately got destroyed in a flood at my old veterinary hospital). In this paper, researchers took beef broth upon which they grew vaccines for humans and infused it with a traceable dye. When the vaccines were eventually given to people, the researchers were able to locate this dye still attached to the protein essence of the beef broth in the lining of the people's intestines. They also found that auto-antibodies were produced that reacted to the foreign beef protein, causing an inflammatory reaction. The paper concluded that what the vaccines are grown on may play a huge role in the cause of irritable bowel syndrome. At this time, inflammatory bowel disease (IBD) was becoming epidemic in dogs and cats, and I postulated that perhaps the cause was the autoimmune reactions caused by the protein tissue upon which we grow vaccines.

Lo and behold, a few years after my first book was published, I received two clinical studies. In the first study, Purdue University's Dr. Larry Glickman and his team found that autoantibodies are formed to a number of different tissues—such as thyroid and connective tissue—after every vaccination.[13] It's thought that the bovine proteins in the vaccines trigger this effect. In the other study, Dr. Michael Lappin at Colorado State University found that vaccination with the feline distemper vaccine—which is grown in a culture of feline kidney cells—creates autoantibodies to kidney tissue.[14] According to Dr. Lappin, the result may be low-grade, but chronic, inflammation in the kidneys. This has long been known to be a primary mechanism behind chronic renal failure (CRF) in cats. Renal failure is now unfortunately the number one cause of feline death.

When I first graduated from Cornell, many vaccines were grown on chicken embryo cultures. Do you know how much chicken allergy we currently see in veterinary practice? A lot! Coincidentally, chicken is one of the most common ingredients in dog food—and also one of the most common food allergens in dogs.[15] In the next chapter, we do a deep dive into the subject of vaccines.

So now that we have a better understanding of the scope of allergy or autoimmune disease beyond "My dog is allergic to grass, what do I do?," let's look at the proper approach to allergy remediation.

If there's suffering—such as severe itching, intense, blood-filled chronic diarrhea, or a potentially fatal acute autoimmune attack on red blood cells or clotting platelets—then conventional medical therapy such as cortisone, antihistamines, or, even stronger, chemotherapy is indicated. However, once stabilization is achieved, our goal is to find a more permanent solution, not suppression of symptoms by chronic drugs that have more side effects than the condition itself.

I have found that food allergies can play a significant role in keeping allergy conditions ongoing. Our practice has derived much benefit from running food-allergy panels, although not 100 percent accurate, based on blood samples sent to a reliable testing laboratory. However, probably the most accurate way of determining if and what your animal companion is allergic to is good old trial and error. You accomplish this by eliminating all proteins except one, whether it's chicken, fish, turkey, bison, or some other animal product. You feed only that one protein for a while and see if your animal companion reacts. If so, then you've got the culprit and you know that you should not feed your companion animal that protein. If not, then you add a second meat protein to the mix or change over to it for a while and again see what happens. In this way, you will eventually determine what animal protein or proteins trigger a reaction.

My favorite nutraceuticals in helping treat and reverse allergy conditions include the natural sterol beta-sitosterol, which is derived from many different plants. The antioxidant quercetin has a powerful antihistamine mast-cell-stabilizing effect. The herb stinging nettle has a Benadryl-like effect without the negative, tranquilizing action of the actual drug. High-quality fish or krill oil, or other high-quality sources of omega-3 fats, in doses above routine maintenance—even up to bowel tolerance—have been proven to have a pronounced anti-inflammatory, antiallergy effect.

The following comprehensive nutraceutical program would successfully support almost any allergy patient. Working with an integrative veterinarian is highly recommended, especially for proper dosing.

- Quercetin: an ultrapotent natural antioxidant that essentially rewires the body's response to allergens by helping to naturally reduce its production of histamines.
- Nettle leaf extract: a powerful plant extract known to help balance the release of irritating cytokines, which can help soothe eye and skin irritation.
- Plant phytosterols: a naturally derived compound that can help calm overactive histamine response.
- Thymus gland extract: To a large extent, the health of the thymus determines the health of the immune system. Thymus extract can help calm the immune system's response to allergens.

- Juvecol: a dietary compound that harnesses the power of proteoglycans (special protein molecules in salmon skin) to help improve overall skin quality in as little as two weeks.
- Omega-3: an essential fatty acid that helps boost skin's overall moisture levels and helps nourish coats.

DISEASE AND AGING

Many pet parents attribute the illness of their animal companions—and themselves—to the inevitable condition of "getting older." Yes, age is linked to the breakdown of the body. We are born in diapers, grow to adulthood, live our hopefully productive and long lives, start to shrink—going back in diapers (actually Depends)—then leave our lives behind as we cross over to the next realm. However, this process happens way too prematurely in both the human and animal kingdoms.

You may recall number nine on my list of New Principles in the Spirit of Healing: "Disease is not something that just happens to you or your animal companions, but something that you allow to happen, either consciously or unconsciously." I know this well because I have witnessed thousands of older patients with fairly bad conditions who then appear and act much younger than their years would lead you to believe when they have received the proper support and guidance.

But age is without a doubt one factor in the wear and tear and breakdown of the body's cells, and it should be taken into account. I try hard to educate pet parents on accepting the physical travail that their animal companions endure on this planet because often they just can't. I'll often hear, "She *can't* have a lump—she's never had one before." My answer to them is "He couldn't have had a heart attack. He never had one before!" That usually does the trick, and they get it.

Then I'll go one step further and try to turn the situation into a positive for them: "Do you know why she now has a lump?"

When they don't know the answer, I respond, "Because she's still here with us!" I call it the Mick Jagger Syndrome—in the words of that classic song "Mother's Little Helper," "What a drag it is getting old!"

And with this I have learned the importance of proactively educating pet parents to start expecting things to happen. Not so much to look for these things, but to accept them as part of the natural aging. When my grandfather was in his late eighties, he used to talk to telephone poles. What could we do? We accepted it and allowed it to be. Who knows— maybe he knew something we didn't!

When I studied with Dr. Bernard Jensen, he taught me one important aspect of natural aging that he learned when he lived with and observed a tribe of people in northern Pakistan called the Hunzas. They lived on food grown in glacial wash-out soil, rarely experienced any disease, and lived to a very old age. What he learned was that these people were robust and active their entire lives, and when their life was coming to its end, they literally stopped working, shriveled up, and passed rapidly. I have used this to educate the moms and dads of pets that live very long lives—into their late teens and even into their twenties. When these dogs and cats suddenly appear to fall apart, and the pet parents don't understand why, it's because that's the way it should be. This is contrary to the current norm in our society—be it humans or animals—to degenerate, suffer, and die over a good portion of our latter days. We are kept "OK" by unnatural means, including drugs, painkillers, and artificial body parts.

I would like to share one last piece of advice on disease treatment. We have well accepted the cause-and-effect relationship that the right treatment is going to elicit a favorable response, and, we hope, quickly. But with true healing, even though we would always like to see that positive and even rapid response, the rule of thumb is that the first thing you want to see when starting a program of support is *change*. And my fundamental rule here is "Any change is better than no change, even if it may appear as a downturn."

Think about it. When a drug addict first comes off an addictive substance, how does he or she typically feel? Horrible, to say the least. Why? Because the body is detoxifying! I have done so much to regain and maintain my health by becoming a runner. So many times, especially after overindulging several days in a row, I do a five- or six-mile run and am left feeling wiped out. But, just a day or two later, I feel back to my old self—before the imbibing.

And one more thing to consider: As animals age and become generally or systemically weak, this will commonly manifest first in the rear legs. I have seen countless pets come in and their parents think the pets have a rear-leg problem. But it's not. This is because the center of gravity is not in the center of their bodies. If you were to put a fulcrum in the middle of a dog or cat's body and try to balance the animal, it wouldn't work because the head is heavier than the tail. They would obviously tip forward. The center of gravity of a four-legged animal is somewhere just behind the shoulder. So, the rear legs are farther from this center than the front, which is why a general weakness will usually present first as a problem with the rear legs.

When I see this and explain it to my clients, I ask them, "What is this called in humans?" No one tracks with me because my answer is "I'm dragging my ass!" Never once have I heard a person who is wiped out say, "I'm dragging my arms!"

AUTOIMMUNE THYROIDITIS

I wrote a section on thyroid disease in my first book, then mentioned autoimmune thyroiditis in a footnote at the section's end. However, this disease is so important to canine health that I feel it is worth mentioning and refining again. Simply stated, in this condition the body makes antibodies against its own thyroid gland, causing it to eventually burn out. The thyroid is like the carburetor of the engine of a car and is centrally vital to both metabolic and hormonal functions of the body.

This is typically a disease of younger dogs, but if left undiagnosed and unaddressed, it can negatively affect dogs throughout their lives. Also, science links vaccinations to this condition as a cause. As mentioned in my first book, one of the most common signs of this disease is behavioral issues. Typical clinical signs include unprovoked aggression toward other animals and/or people, sudden onset of seizure disorder in adulthood, disorientation, moodiness, erratic temperament, periods of hyperactivity, hypo-attentiveness, depression, fearfulness and phobias, anxiety, submissiveness, passivity, compulsiveness, and/or irritability.[16]

If a dog has this condition—and especially marked behavioral problems—in my experience it will be extremely difficult to improve this patient's behavior and quality of life without first addressing this thyroid condition. However, if properly diagnosed and treated, the positive behavioral changes can be dramatic.

The only proper way to diagnosis this condition is by way of extensive thyroid blood tests. It has also been my experience, seeing so many thousands of dogs in my career, that veterinarians do not, unfortunately, sufficiently and properly test thyroid function. And when they do, it's usually to add just one thyroid test, called a T4, to routine blood work. According to Dr. Jean Dodds, *the* expert on thyroid disease in our profession and the veterinarian who has done the most work and publishing on autoimmune thyroiditis, "Evaluating a dog's thyroid function based solely on a T4 is useless!"

I have seen many dogs over the decades—especially those with behavioral issues, allergies, and other chronic problems—get worlds better when we have diagnosed and properly addressed autoimmune thyroiditis in them that had gone undetected. Remember, however, that this form of thyroid disease is heritable, so these dogs should not be used for breeding, and their parents and siblings need to be screened annually for thyroiditis—for the sake of their own health and for suitability for breeding.

I have also seen quite a few young dogs who appear to be healthy, but when we do extensive thyroid testing just once—when we do their routine blood work—we find that their autoimmune thyroid levels are quite elevated. Then by properly treating this, we have literally saved their lives.

So, as a routine—especially in younger dogs—I highly recommend that when blood samples are taken to add in a comprehensive thyroid panel consisting of at least a T4, Free T4, T3, and a thyroglobulin autoantibody test. To do it completely, you can also have T3 and T4 autoantibody tests added.

While we're on this subject, I have been bothered by and have tried so hard to educate on one thing over the years. That's the veterinarian who makes a decision for a patient's lifetime based on just one result—one point in time. As much as I have done much of my patient guidance based upon blood results, as it's the true reflection of the patient at a particular moment, I also realize that the body is in constant flux. That is why there are normal reference "ranges" for blood results. You can wake in the morning and your blood sugar can be in the low sixties, then test it again after dinner and it can be in the high nineties.

I guarantee that your liver enzymes have not been "normal" every day of your life. To prove that, go to a wedding on a Saturday night and just have a great time. Then go to your doctor on Tuesday and have your blood tested. Even better, go run the New York City Marathon, then check yourself into a hospital saying you are feeling wiped out, not saying anything about the marathon. Chances are, some of your blood results will indicate that you are critically ill.

And then there is the possibility of lab error. I unfortunately had to learn this lesson at the beginning of my career. I had just graduated from veterinary school and got my first job in Horseheads, New York. Suddenly, I was no longer attached to my parents' apron strings and needed to get my own insurance policy. The company requested a full physical exam. I established a relationship with a highly recommended MD. I went in for the exam and had full blood samples taken. They made an appointment for me the next Tuesday to come in to go over everything and write me the necessary forms. I called the office on Monday to confirm my appointment, and they immediately put the doctor on the phone, which I thought a bit strange.

The doctor said that he knew I was coming in the next day and he figured this could possibly wait, but since I was on the phone, he would take the opportunity to talk with me. Getting a bit freaked-out, I asked, "What's up?"

"According to your blood results, you are either going into early kidney failure, or you have a tumor on your parathyroid gland, or . . ."

I was in shock. What could the *third* option be?

The third option was lab error.

Now, I thought, what was the chance that one of the largest medical labs in the country would make an error of that magnitude?

The doctor asked if I could come over and repeat the blood tests. I was there in eight minutes! He rushed the tests through, and on Tuesday I got the results: all was normal! Sometimes we do just have to learn the hard way.

BLITZ AND ME

The greatest pleasure I get from being a veterinarian is when, against seemingly hopeless odds, I return an ill animal companion back to health—sometimes one that is on death's doorstep. While the gratitude of a happy pet parent is the icing on the cake, the long-term well-being of the cake (the animal companion) is what's most important to me.

When Lance Fargo of Millville, Delaware, brought Blitz—his young, field-competition Weimaraner—to me, the dog was in bad shape. When Blitz was just nine months old, he was injured in a twelve-foot fall onto a concrete patio. About a year and a half later, Blitz's diaphragm was found to have a hernia, which required surgery to repair. After that, he suffered from an abscessed lung. Removing the abscess necessitated a second surgery, during which most of one of his lungs was removed. Both these surgeries were performed at veterinary-university hospitals.

Says Lance Fargo about Blitz's condition after the second surgery:

> While he was recovering from that, he was very frail and weak. And I took him back up, and they found an infection in his chest that was literally eating away the bone in his chest. Surgically, they tried to clean it out three times—but, finally, the doctor told me

there wasn't anything else he could do and recommended euthanizing him.[17]

That's when, in 2005, Lance brought Blitz to me to try to save his life. I kept Blitz for four days, and we administered IV vitamin C to bolster his immune system. Then I returned him to Lance—telling him that Blitz would eventually be able to return to his normal activities, but not to rush it.

Blitz recovered fully—with the exception of that missing lung—and a grateful pet parent gave me something to be proud of: a beautiful bronze plaque with the following text:

It is with extreme gratitude that Lance Fargo and his best friend Blitz present this plaque to Dr. Marty for his critical efforts in saving Blitz's life. In the fall of 2004, Blitz, one of the most promising young field competition Weimaraners in the country, was suffering from a highly aggressive and life-threatening infection. All attempts to save Blitz through traditional veterinary medicine failed. Finally, Blitz visited with Dr. Marty in a last-ditch effort to save his life. Dr. Marty successfully reversed Blitz's deteriorating health and saved him from certain death. In 2007, after two years of rehabilitation and training, Blitz returned to field competition. He finished the year ranked as the #4 Field Trial Weimaraner in the country. On March 15, 2008, Blitz completed his quest for the AKC title "FIELD CHAMPION" by winning the Open Gun Dog stake at the Eastern German Shorthaired Pointer Club's Spring Field

Trial. We could not have achieved this accomplishment without the intervening and healing hand of Dr. Marty. Well done Blitz. Well done Dr. Marty.

ASK DR. MARTY

Q: With all the advances in science, I don't understand why our animal companions still get cancer and other deadly diseases. What is the overall state of health and disease in the animals we love so much?

A: After being in this profession for almost half a century, I see clearly that the smarter we get, the more we learn, and the greater our advancements, the less healthy we and our animal companions are. Sure, the life expectancy of humans has increased, but I wonder at what loss in the quality of life. Look around, and you'll see that many older people are still with us because of the use of artificial or transplanted body parts and dramatic medical interventions. At the same time, life quality has diminished as the symptoms that we would normally exhibit are being chemically suppressed. There is just no doubt that cancer and other chronic, degenerative illnesses have steadily increased in our companion animals despite advances in the field of medicine. I believe we need to step back, take a fresh look at the situation, and come up with another game plan for health care. Our current, big-business-dominated system is unsustainable—and it results in less than optimal medical outcomes for those we love.

ELSA'S STORY

When Steve brought his Staffordshire terrier—aka a pit bull—Elsa to me, she had squamous cell carcinoma of the tonsil that had spread to her lymph node. The lymph node and the tonsil were originally both removed at Long Island Veterinary Specialists—LIVS. Squamous cell carcinoma in this same location is the cancer that killed actor Sammy Davis Jr.

When the results were received by LIVS, they told Steve that the cancer was beyond their scope and they could do nothing. They referred him to the Animal Medical Center— AMC. The oncologist there gave Steve a poor prognosis and said, "If you don't use chemotherapy, expect things to start popping out all over within six weeks. With chemotherapy, she's got five months to live if we're lucky."

So, Steve came up to Smith Ridge for a consult—in those days, it was a little over an hour's drive. I talked with Steve as I do with all my new clients, showed him before-and-after photos of many successful patients, and all the rest. Not once did he look up. I kept talking and talking—most people start to smile after a while. Not Steve.

After about half an hour, I just looked at him and asked, "What are you doing here?"

"What do you mean?"

"I asked 'What are you doing here?' because you're obviously not interested in anything I'm saying."

"Truthfully, my girlfriend found you online, and if I didn't come, she would kill me!"

While I don't remember exactly how I said it, I kind of

went off on Steve—telling him what a waste of a human being he was. I struck a nerve in him. All of a sudden, with tears streaming down his face, he looked up at me and said, "I still think my dog is going to die, but I want to thank you because you just saved *my* life. I became so despondent that I lost all faith in everything."

Steve ended up with Elsa when he and his ex-wife were walking down a street in Brooklyn and they found Elsa tied to a tree. Steve didn't like dogs. The wife took Elsa home and they adopted her. When they broke up, because Steve had fallen so in love with Elsa, he kept her.

After Steve told me about how he had lost faith in everything, he walked around the desk and hugged me and thanked me for saving his life. I looked at him and said, "You just wasted thirty-five minutes of a one-hour consult. Do you want to work on your dog?"

"Let's go for it!"

We already had a double confirmation on Elsa's tumor, first by LIVS and then AMC. Because of the aggressiveness of the tumor, I put Elsa on a load of supplements; I believe it was up to eleven different ones. Steve went home and became a monster. He researched and added in twenty-eight more supplements a day. He hired two professional chefs. He was importing organic salmon from Norway and buying organic filet mignon for Elsa. He was spending around $10,000 to $12,000 a month on therapy for Elsa, and he was driving from Long Island to Smith Ridge—about an hour and twenty minutes each way—at least every four or five days to have Elsa examined.

About three months after we started, I examined Elsa—

looking down her throat. I could see that the cancer had returned to the area where the tonsil had been removed. I sedated Elsa, took a biopsy for testing, then photographed the tumor. I performed a fifteen-minute cryosurgery to kill the cancer. The results soon came back from the testing: squamous cell carcinoma. So, now I had triple confirmation.

It was approaching Christmas and Steve decided to throw a party to celebrate the five-month anniversary of when the oncologist had told him Elsa would be dead. He invited everyone whose lives were touched by Elsa, and who had touched Elsa's life, which was around ninety-five people. He took over a huge Italian restaurant on the water in Long Beach, Long Island. He had unlimited Dom Pérignon champagne available and invited me to say a few words, which I happily did.

Then, Elsa's godfather—actor Chazz Palminteri—gave the anti-eulogy for her. I had Steve and Chazz on my third SiriusXM radio show, and Chazz announced, "I just want everyone to know that, ten years ago, I had cancer of the throat. I'm still alive because of the support and hope and Steve coming to the hospital—combined with the proper therapy."

Fast-forward to the six-and-a-half-month mark. I looked down Elsa's throat and the cancer had returned once again. This showed that surgery doesn't cure cancer; it often just buys you time to work on the immune system. However, despite the cancer, Elsa was still doing fine clinically. So, I did another biopsy and photographed the tumor. The results came back, and it was squamous cell carcinoma. There's no way anyone could say the tumor had been misdiagnosed—we had quadruple confirmation.

Using cryosurgery, I froze this tumor, and Elsa lived cancer-free for *nine* more years.

All that time later, Elsa was getting old. She was drinking and urinating a lot—symptoms that maybe Elsa's kidneys were failing. This was confirmed by their local veterinarian. Steve called and said, "I want to bring her up to Smith Ridge."

"Sure, no problem," I said. So, we had it all planned for Steve and Elsa to come up—I think it was on a Wednesday. But, two days before Steve was supposed to bring Elsa to Smith Ridge, his mother died. So, we postponed the appointment a day. And in that one day, the biggest hurricane to ever hit Long Island—Hurricane Sandy—wiped out his entire area. His local veterinary clinic was taken out, so he didn't have access to any veterinary medicine. There was no gas and he couldn't get to Smith Ridge—he couldn't get off Long Island.

He got me on the phone, and I promised to get him fluids and injectable kidney extracts and a bunch of stuff to help Elsa. But how was I going to get it there? Steve found a FedEx truck driver and gave him a whole load of money. If I would send the medications via FedEx, this guy would find the package and personally drive it over to Steve's place on Long Island. Steve set up a mini-clinic in his house, and we started to treat Elsa. She lived another seventeen months with great quality of life despite having total kidney failure.

At one time, Elsa was the only dog in the history of NYU Medical to have her own entry badge. Steve and Elsa had badges to come and go into NYU Medical to visit cancer patients and bring them hope. In her latter stages, when she couldn't travel any longer, NYU Medical sent cancer patients to Steve's house in Long Beach to meet Elsa for hope.

Illustrated children's books are now being written about Elsa's life, and Steve's brother—a cinematographer—is working on a documentary about her. It's such an amazing story, and it changed Steve's life forever.

It's said that 85 to 90 percent of the activity of our brains is beyond our conscious awareness. So, if you take that vibration and put it at the vibrational level of thought, which I'm sure has the same electromagnetic spectrum of vibration, you turn a person's feeling of hopelessness and despair and sadness into one of joy and hope. And all of a sudden, the person's pet is getting better. The mind is a powerful thing. Hope springs eternal. In many cases, as I wrote in the third New Principle in the Spirit of Healing, "Hope consistently precedes healing."

A little over a decade ago, *The New York Times* published an excellent article about the implications of doctors who take hope away from patients. According to the article, titled "When Doctors Steal Hope," when a doctor gives a patient an extremely poor prognosis—putting patient and loved ones into premature grief—the doctor steals away the emotional energy they need to support the patient through what may well turn out to be a long and difficult recovery.

Why do so many doctors and veterinarians give the very worst news when the future is uncertain? Says one doctor quoted in the article, "In some ways it's easier to give people the worst news, and then if something good comes about, everyone is overjoyed."[18]

While I agree that the duty of veterinarians is to be transparent and truthful with pet parents and patients alike, I don't believe it's their job to steal hope. I know it's not. The unfortunate thing is that so many veterinarians—unaware of the incredible potential of alternative therapies to create positive responses in cases that appear hopeless—don't know any better. So, their giving poor prognoses is what is true for them. This just may be the top priority for the rest of my life regarding my profession: to educate about and bring forth these therapies.

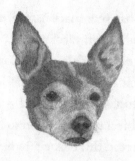

8

DOCTOR, DO NO HARM

Sooner or later everyone sits down to a
banquet of their consequences.
—ROBERT LOUIS STEVENSON

This was a difficult chapter for me to write. Every veterinarian I know has joined this profession out of an immense amount of love and caring for the dogs, cats, and other companion animals concerned pet parents bring to us every day. Most of us have companion animals of our own—often many—and we love them as if they are a part of our families. However, the veterinary establishment has trained us to do things that sometimes bring harm to the very animals we have promised to protect, and that is where I have to draw the line in my own practice.

While more than a few areas of conventional veterinary medicine ultimately do more harm than good, I believe the number one way that veterinarians can routinely harm our animal companions is with vaccinations.

I wrote an entire chapter on vaccinations in my first book, and my intent is not to duplicate what I've already written. However, so much has changed in this area over the past twenty years that I feel the obligation to bring that material up-to-date. As you read this chapter, remember that I am not anti-vaccine—I am pro-sanity.

THE SCOURGE OF OVERVACCINATION

Decades ago, my dear colleagues and vaccine experts Professor Ron Schultz and Dr. Jean Dodds were among the few people saying—along with me—that we were overvaccinating pets. I was called irresponsible in public at a large veterinary conference because others were unwilling to consider that vaccines might not always be needed or safe for dogs and cats. Today, a lot of people are still shooting arrows at us even though our backs are full of them! All joking aside, despite the criticism, we were and remain determined to continue to educate the public and pet parents around the world about this critically important topic.

Dr. Ron Schultz—professor emeritus at the University of Wisconsin School of Veterinary Medicine—is one of the people who has pushed for taking a more balanced approach to analyzing the risks and benefits of vaccines for individual animals before administering them. In a presentation of scientific papers on vaccines, he explained the two laws of statistics:

- The first law of statistics: if the statistics don't support your viewpoint, you obviously need more statistics.
- The second law of statistics: given enough statistics, you can prove anything.

As Professor Schultz says, "Be wise and immunize, but immunize wisely!"

Edward Jenner developed the first scientifically proven smallpox vaccine by using cowpox as the inoculum in 1796, although the approach was used privately by farmer Benjamin Jesty in 1774 to protect his family from smallpox. Ever since, vaccines have been used commercially and for research in humans and animals to elicit protective immunity to specific infectious agents. Despite these long-standing efforts and focus on vaccine-related issues, this subject remains one of the most contentious of all human and animal medical safety and efficacy procedures.

Many veterinary practitioners simply believe what they have been taught about vaccines and so are less inclined to change or "fix" what is perceived to be unbroken. However, to other veterinarians, canine vaccination programs have been "practice management tools"—business profit centers—rather than medical procedures. Not surprisingly, therefore, attempts to change the vaccines and vaccination programs based on scientific information have created significant controversy. Unfortunately, a more-is-better philosophy still prevails with regard to pet vaccines.

Routine, calendar-generated vaccination has been and remains the single most important reason why most pet parents bring their pets to a veterinarian for an annual or, more often, a "wellness" visit. Another reason for the reluctance to change current vaccination programs is the failure to understand the principles of vaccinal immunity (that portion of immunity conveyed by vaccines). Clearly, the accumulated evidence indicates that vaccination protocols should no longer be considered a one-size-fits-all program.

Even today, estimates are that only about 40 percent of veterinarians are following the current, standardized vaccine policy guidelines put forth by the highest organizations in the profession.* There is no such thing as an "up-to-date" or "due" vaccination. Enlightened veterinarians can now offer a package of separated vaccine components, when available, rather than give them all together, since the published data show more adverse reactions when multiple vaccines are administered at the same time.

Summary on Vaccine Policy

AAHA, 2003

Current knowledge supports the statement:

- No vaccine is always safe, no vaccine is always protective, and no vaccine is always indicated.

---

* WSAVA—World Small Animal Veterinary Association; AVMA—American Veterinary Medical Association; AAHA—American Animal Hospital Association; BVA—British Veterinary Association.

WSAVA, 2015–17

From Professor Michael J. Day:

- Vaccination should be just one part of a holistic preventive health care program for pets that is most simply delivered within the framework of an annual health check consultation.
- Vaccination is an act of veterinary science that should be considered as individualized medicine, tailored for the needs of the individual pet, and delivered as one part of a preventive medicine program in an annual health check visit.

But vaccines also contain a variety of additives and adjuvants that can increase the risk of adverse reactions to the shots. It's important to know something about these additional ingredients, to talk to your veterinarian about any concerns, and to help protect your pet by avoiding unnecessary vaccination whenever possible.

Vaccines are not innocuous products, so the benefit/risk equation needs to be assessed before vaccination, even for rabies in unhealthy pets.

WHAT ABOUT VACCINE DOSE AND PET WEIGHT AND SIZE?

One ongoing concern about overvaccination in dogs is the giving of vaccines on a one-size-fits-all basis rather than based upon the body weight of the animal. Why do toy-breed (for example, a Chihuahua) and giant-breed dogs (such as a Great Dane) receive the exact same dose?

They routinely do.

This is especially puzzling when you consider that the manufacturer's vaccine clinical trials are typically performed on laboratory beagles with little field testing in different dog breeds prior to licensure and clinical use. Surely, a giant-breed dog should require more vaccine than a small- or medium-size dog to fully immunize, and toy and smaller breeds would logically need less.

ASK DR. MARTY

Q: Whether to vaccinate has become one of biggest controversies in both human and animal medical practice. What's your take on this?

A: In basic theory, I am against vaccinations, but as you might have heard me say in the documentary film *The Dog Doc,* "I am not anti-vaccination—I am pro-sanity!" Isaac Newton's third law of motion, formulated in 1686, states that for every action there is an equal and opposite reaction. We are all given an immune system that should function optimally when unadulterated. So, if you artificially and powerfully stimulate one aspect of it, some other aspect of it needs to decline. I believe there is a direct link between how we've come to vaccinate companion animals and the higher-than-ever incidence of chronic, degenerative illness—especially cancer. We cannot make immune systems bionic and function at a level higher than 100 percent across the board—it's just not possible.

Because we humans have over the centuries tipped the scales of health more in favor of disease, we have created the apparent need for vaccinations. My concern with our animal companions is that this has become a runaway train of insanity. We've accepted that pets need all their vaccinations, often annually, given all at the same time, and in doses that are identical in strength—the same for a Great Dane and a Chihuahua. And vaccinations are even administered to animals of ill health because "they're due," despite the warning literature included with vaccines that states that they should be given only to healthy animals.

Every veterinarian should carefully consider when and in what dosages the dogs and cats in his or her care receive vaccinations. We also need scientific studies applied to the dose-to-weight relationship for appropriate administration to properly assist veterinarians. Vaccination should be a considered step and not just automatic. Hippocrates said it all: "First, do no harm!"

DURATION OF IMMUNITY FROM VACCINES

The "core" vaccines given to, in most cases, dogs and cats confer long-lived (even lifelong) immunity once the initial puppy or kitten series is completed, and with some, singly boosted. However, this is typically accepted as a three-year duration, after which boosters are still typically given even though serum antibody titers (a blood test to assess the level of immunity an animal has) can be measured instead to assess the existing level of protection.

For rabies vaccines, after the initial two doses are given within twelve months, boosters are required every three years. The recently completed Rabies Challenge Fund studies determined that the rabies vaccine conveyed protection after live rabies virus challenge in dogs for five years (www .rabieschallengefund.org).

Most of the pets we test for immunity to rabies in our practice—blood serum samples are sent to Kansas State University (KSU) Veterinary Diagnostic Laboratory, the gold standard, for analysis—have titers demonstrating immunity way above what is considered acceptable even by the World Health Organization for import/export in the United States. Just for example, I would like to share one case here that I present when I lecture, even to veterinary colleges—a sixty-six-pound Weimaraner named Ocean.

Ocean came to me as a puppy, already weighing in his sixties, and he had experienced a bad reaction to his earlier puppy vaccines. His mom was concerned about giving him his first rabies vaccine. Although a rabies shot is legally mandated and given at full dose, the same for all pets, I was also concerned. So, I decided to give Ocean a fraction of the dose, just to test the waters. If there was no reaction, I would then give the proper dose a few weeks later. Also, out of curiosity, I wanted to send a blood sample to KSU to test his immunity.

Because Ocean's pet parents lived some distance from

Smith Ridge, they did not make it back for months. They were willing to start with sending that titer to KSU, followed by the proper vaccination. When that titer came back, any ratio equal to or greater than 1:5 was considered to be acceptable for humans by the WHO. Ocean's ratio was higher than 1:7,000! Based on his previous negative vaccine reaction, coupled with this scientific evidence, we wrote a medical exemption that was accepted.

Routine titers continued.

Next was 1:5,300—still far above the WHO recommended ratio. Three years later, KSU changed their parameters, and in writing—which I present in my talks—published that a value equal to or greater than 0.1 IU/ml is considered "protection" in pets. Ocean's came back greater than 15. That is a 150-fold increase over the acceptable level. Those values continued the rest of his life, and when he reached older age in his teens, weighing nearly eighty pounds, it remained 44 times higher than 0.1 IU/ml.

I also found a scientific study performed in Uganda on humans between the ages of two and nineteen years. They were properly vaccinated for a strain of meningitis, then properly tested for acceptable immunity. The results showed that vaccines given at one-half, and down to one-fifth, the usual dose imparted lasting immunity. Only the dose given at one-tenth the usual dose was not adequate. But the conclusion of the study was *not* to just use lower doses. Instead, the study stated that, during emergencies, less than the full dose can be given—down to one-fifth usual dosage—to enable more people to be vaccinated with a limited amount of vaccine available. I don't understand this logic.

WHAT ARE VACCINE ADDITIVES AND ADJUVANTS?

These ingredients include the carrier molecules and immune stimulants (that is, the adjuvants) that are intended to improve the efficacy of vaccines. They also include excipients—the inactive ingredients in vaccines that are present in only small amounts. They are preservatives such as thimerosal (mercury) to prevent contamination, stabilizers (such as sugars or gelatin) to preserve vaccines during storage and transport, and adjuvants such as the salts from such metals as aluminum and mercury.

Adjuvants accelerate, prolong, or enhance the immune response when used together with specific vaccine antigens (for example, the viral proteins of infectious diseases). But adjuvants also increase the risk of adverse autoimmune and inflammatory events following vaccination.

Finally, vaccines also contain residual trace amounts of the cell culture materials used to grow the antigens, such as egg protein, human serum albumin, fetal calf serum, yeast proteins, and other culture media. They may also contain ingredients such as formaldehyde—used to kill viruses and inactivate toxins—and antibiotics (for example, neomycin and gentamicin) to prevent bacterial contamination.

WHAT KINDS OF ADVERSE EFFECTS ARE KNOWN?

Adjuvants have been used relatively safely in human and veterinary medicine for decades, but the debate and controversy about their efficacy versus their safety is not expected to be resolved in the foreseeable future.

Adjuvants can produce numerous adverse effects. But because vaccines are viewed as inherently safe and nontoxic, toxicity studies are often excluded from the regulatory safety assessment of vaccines. Young animals are especially at risk as they are more vulnerable to toxicity than adults and are regularly exposed to more adjuvants with the typical vaccination series they receive as puppies and kittens.

Adjuvants impact the central nervous system at all levels and can do so by changing expression of the individual's genes. Further, adjuvants are now known to strongly affect the nervous system / immune axis, which plays a key role in brain development and immune function.

The autoimmune (auto-inflammatory) syndrome induced by adjuvants (ASIA syndrome) was first defined in 2011.[1] Presently, it includes four conditions that share similar signs and symptoms, one of which is from the effects of vaccination. The common denominator in these syndromes is the triggering effect of adjuvants, in combination with other environmental factors along with genetic predisposition. When combined, these factors cause the failure of self-tolerance, which equates to autoimmunity.

Heavy metals such as mercury and aluminum are directly involved as well, especially in the thimerosal-preserved (mercury-preserved) canine rabies vaccines. The allergy or immune response induced by these metals is a delayed-type hypersensitivity that begins around three days but can occur up to forty-five days after vaccination. It often manifests as contact dermatitis (skin inflammation), liver or joint damage, seizures, aggression, phobias, or an attack on the red blood cells and/or platelets. This is the allergic breakthrough phenomenon, which I mentioned in chapter 7.

In his keynote speech at the Truth About Cancer Live 2019, Robert Kennedy Jr. explained that adjuvants enhance the potency of the organism in vaccines. We used to vaccinate with modified live viruses, which are known as MLVs, but they were becoming virulent in the body. So we switched to killed-virus vaccines. However, they weren't stimulating as much of an immune response, so adjuvants were added to enhance the immunological response. Kennedy said that two of the most powerful neurotoxins aside from radiation are mercury and aluminum.

So many of the problems we're seeing are not just the result of vaccine potencies that can be up to ten times what's required for a Great Dane; they're the result of these other ingredients that are a part of vaccines. And the adjuvants are probably at the top of the heap.

In my first book, I wrote about the insanity of what's called the *feline vaccine-induced fibrosarcoma*. In certain cases, where the vaccine enters a cat's body, the cat grows a fibrosarcoma. The rabies vaccine is typically implicated, but the feline leukemia shot has also been considered. No matter how many times you surgically remove it cleanly, the tumor grows back with a vengeance and will most likely kill the cat.

One of the number one veterinary oncologists in the United States is Dr. Philip Bergman, director of clinical studies for VCA Animal Hospitals. He's the guy that the big pharmaceutical companies hire to create chemotherapeutics to treat cancer. I went to a continuing-education presentation that he gave about the feline vaccine-induced fibrosarcoma. The only way to prevent regrowth of this tumor besides amputating the affected part (which cannot be done because most vaccines are still given between the shoulder blades) is to remove the tumor with five-centimeter margins. In the cat that he showed undergoing the procedure, this means cutting off the tops of both shoulder blades and the tops of five of the backbones. Then you sew the cat up. It's a barbaric procedure.

Then he said, "This is not a disease solution from surgery; this is a disease caused solely by the adjuvants." And they did a study and proved it.[2] Dr. Bergman explained that the only solution is for veterinarians to buy and administer adjuvant-free vaccines.

HOW PREVALENT ARE ADVERSE REACTIONS TO VACCINE INGREDIENTS?

Both veterinary practitioners and pet caregivers are seeing more animals exhibiting signs of immune dysfunction and disease—such things as difficulty breathing, diarrhea, increased heart rate, weakness, shock, and even death—many of which occur within thirty to forty-five days of a vaccination. Vaccines and their adjuvants are implicated as the potential triggering agents in animals genetically predisposed to adverse vaccine reactions, a problem termed *vaccinosis*.

USING SERUM ANTIBODY TITERS INSTEAD OF BOOSTERS FOR IMMUNIZED PETS

In the intervening years between booster vaccinations, and in the case of geriatric pets, circulating humoral immunity can be evaluated by measuring serum vaccine antibody titers as an indication of the presence of immune memory. Simply put, if we can test that an animal has evidence of enough protection in his bloodstream against a certain disease, say distemper, then shouldn't that be a more reliable indicator if the individual is due for a vaccine than a calendar?

Unfortunately, taking titers is more time-consuming and more expensive to the pet parents than simply giving the vaccine, so that becomes an easy selling point for the veterinarian in support of giving routine shots. As true as this may be, remember the pitch in that old Fram oil filter ad with the auto mechanic holding up the filter and saying, "Pay me now or pay me later." Spending just a little more preventively could save patient suffering and thousands of dollars in medical expenses if an adverse reaction to a vaccine leads to a deeper, chronic illness.

HOW GOVERNMENT GETS INVOLVED

Government can and often has played an important role in promoting the health and wellness of both people and their animal companions. However, sometimes government gets it wrong. In the case of people, this is clearly the case in California, which passed a new vaccine law that went into effect on January 1, 2020. Among other things, the law removed the final authority for vaccine medical exemptions from doctors and placed this authority with the California Department of Public Health.

While doctors will still be able to write vaccination waiver letters for children who are considered to be at risk, doctors who write five or more such waiver letters in one year will be reviewed by the California Department of Public Health. If the department determines that the doctor is "contributing to a public health risk," then he or she will be reported to the state medical board for further investigation and possible sanction, during which time waivers written by that doctor will be canceled.

The result is that children with valid medical reasons to avoid the fifteen or more vaccines required just to enter kindergarten in California will be given the shots anyway. Doctors will likely decide that it's not worth risking their licenses over the issue.

And make no mistake about it, vaccines and children are an issue. According to the Centers for Disease Control and Prevention (CDC), vaccinations in humans can and do sometimes have negative side effects. For example, the most recent vaccine information statement posted on the CDC website in August 2019 for the MMR (measles, mumps, and rubella) vaccine states that possible negative reactions include fever, seizures, pneumonia, swelling of the brain and/or spinal cord covering, and infection that may be life-threatening in people with serious immune system problems.[3]

According to an article published by CalMatters, a nonpartisan, nonprofit journalism website that tracks regulation, education, health care, and other issues in California:

> In 1986, the federal government created the National Childhood Vaccine Injury Act that freed pharmaceutical companies from liability in cases of such injury. Under that law, billions of government dollars have been paid to families with children harmed by vaccines.[4]

At a press conference after California governor Gavin Newsom signed the new vaccine bill into law in September 2019, Robert F. Kennedy Jr. asked, "Where are the legal and rational boundaries now that the government can force a medical procedure on children?"[5]

Good question.

At the Truth About Cancer Live 2019, Robert Kennedy Jr. explained the other effects this California bill would have on the state's citizens. Four thousand children had documented bad reactions to vaccinations who subsequently received medical exemptions from their family MDs. These exemptions then became invalid unless the reaction was anaphylaxis—or *death*. And if any exemption could be claimed, then it would be only for that *one virus*. The vaccine-sensitive child would be required to get all the other required vaccinations. How barbaric! It's no wonder that I have already heard so many stories of concerned families packing up and moving out of that state.

Dr. Andrew Wakefield so eloquently expressed in his British manner at the same conference how, on this planet, nothing is more sacred than the bond between mother and child, and the mother's intuition that goes along with that. With this new law passed in California, moms *know* how much harm will be imparted to their children as they are being legally forced to give them more vaccinations—even after their children have been damaged by previous ones. Where have we come in human society to violate a bond as precious as this?

Finally, I had the honor of being invited to attend the event where Bobby Kennedy Jr. received a lifetime achievement award for the amazing and so valuable humanitarian work toward which he has dedicated his life. I was simply blown away by his acceptance speech, which easily surpassed half an hour. In this talk, he shared the following information: In the 1980s, pharmaceutical companies made at least $250 million on vaccines a year. Now, that figure has increased to $50 billion, and they generate $500 billion from the sale of the drugs that they market to treat the epidemic of childhood diseases caused by their vaccines.

So what does all this have to do with our animal companions? Why should we concern ourselves with the vaccine industry's power over humans? Unfortunately, the situation is even worse for animals. While most humans stop getting vaccinated after childhood—with the exception of tetanus boosters every ten years and seasonal flu vaccines, which are recommended, but optional—it's different for dogs and cats. Vaccinations are required (for rabies) and recommended for some diseases, in most cases at least every three years, until the day the pets die—or are caused to become ill and die.

In January 2020, Maggie's Vaccine Protection Act, formally known as House Bill 214, passed the Delaware General Assembly. Previously, Delaware law required all dogs to be given vaccines regardless of their physical condition or health. Under Maggie's Vaccine Protection Act—named for a shih tzu that died due to overvaccination in 2016—veterinarians will be allowed to use titers to determine whether a dog, cat, or other animal companion needs the vaccines.

Said Delaware state senator Gerald Hocker, "Vaccinations will be based on the health of the dog. Who better than the veterinarian to decide, depending on the health of the dog?"[6] I agree wholeheartedly with this perspective, and it's my fervent hope that similar laws will soon be passed in other states.

IT'S US AGAINST THEM

During his keynote presentation at the Truth About Cancer Live 2019 conference, Dr. Wakefield explained that our dependence on vaccinations stems at least in part from our perception of microbes as the enemy—dangerous microscopic creatures that are a constant threat to our health and well-being. Without a doubt, our animal companions can and do become infected by bacteria and viruses, and they get sick and sometimes die as a result—the same as we humans. However, I would argue that dogs and cats with healthy immune systems mostly get along just fine with the vast majority of "infectious disease" organisms in their environment.

Now, canine distemper and parvo disease exist and typically aren't mild, but I can count the total number of cases together that I have seen in my entire career on less than two hands. And half of those recovered after intravenous vitamin C therapy. Even if we can attribute a lot of this low incidence to the positive effects of vaccine protocols, I have also seen and treated tens of thousands of cancer patients, and there is clearly a scientific link between vaccines and immune suppression. Even for veterinarians living in areas where the incidence of these two diseases is more prevalent than within my experience, I can guarantee that the amount of cancer they see still tremendously surpasses this. We must take a better look at this scenario.

As I mentioned in chapter 6, one gram—just one twenty-eighth of an ounce—of dog poop typically contains an average 23 million fecal coliform bacteria. When the immune systems of our animal companions are weakened by low-quality food, pesticides, chemicals, drugs, vaccines, and other agents in their environment, they lose their good health and succumb to illness. Not only that, but as Robert Kennedy Jr. pointed out in his keynote at the Truth About Cancer Live 2019, the more diseases beings go through in youth—such as measles, chicken pox, and more in the case of humans—the stronger and more resilient their immune systems are later on in life, and they live longer according to studies that have tracked them.

Herd health is a concept routinely used in the livestock, dairy, and other animal-related industries. As you can imagine, every cattle rancher, dairy farmer, sheepherder, zookeeper, and other person who works with large groups of animals lives in mortal fear of a disease spreading from one animal to another—potentially making them unmarketable or even causing their death. Mothers who are vaccinated do not pass on passive immunity after the initial colostrum milk to their offspring.

The two phases of life when mammals of all sorts are most vulnerable to the diseases we vaccinate them for are in their first year and in old age. In the first few weeks after they are born, mammals rely on the passive immunity they receive from their mothers to protect them. That passive immunity is neutralized if the mother gets vaccinated just before giving birth and typically wanes in the puppies of all vaccinated mothers by twelve to fourteen weeks of age.

As Dr. Andrew Wakefield points out, nature requires balance. The immune system has three arms. One is the antibody arm, which deals with viruses outside the cell—through the blood. So, for example, when a virus is introduced into the bloodstream, antibodies are made against the virus, and these antibodies also circulate in the bloodstream, targeting and killing the virus. The second arm of the immune system is cellular—these are the killer cells that protect against viruses *inside* the cells. The third arm—added to Dr. Wakefield's model by Dr. Jean Dodds—is the secretory immunity in bodily secretions such as saliva, tears, sweat, feces, and urogenital fluids. You need a balance between the three arms of the immune system.

If you concentrate on building immunity through vaccines, you're blowing the antibody arm of the immune system out of proportion—producing a high antibody titer, which is generally considered to be a good outcome in medicine. However, if you pump the body full of vaccines—focusing not on the cellular arm, but on the antibody arm—you get a paradoxical effect in cellular immunity. Low cellular immunity accelerates viral and other microbial growth and mutations. You select a strain of the virus (bacteria or fungus) or the vaccine that doesn't simulate nature—you're doing this artificially.

Then, just like bacteria that become resistant to antibiotics with their overuse, viruses also start to mutate—becoming resistant to everything. Vaccines are creating mutant viruses—overwhelming weak immune systems and causing chronic illness or death. Of course, the last thing we want to do is anything that enhances viral mutation. Think about it. The vaccination industry is one of the few that makes money through failure. The more they fail, the more vaccines they produce, and the more they sell.

Surprisingly, one of the main reasons vaccines have routinely been deemed to be harmless by regulators is that they only trace side effects directly related to the disease that is being vaccinated against. So, for example, if they are testing a vaccine for diphtheria, then they only trace the side effects directly related to that one specific disease: diphtheria. They never look at "unrelated" things, such as the prevalence of cancer, autoimmune disease, and even latent mortality. Also, because vaccines have been deemed inherently safe, toxicity studies are usually not required by government regulatory oversight. This narrow focus, I believe, causes us to miss seeing the forest for the trees.

WHY IS SO MUCH OVERVACCINATION GOING ON?

It was Dr. Dodds who originally taught me that, according to USDA studies, the vaccines we routinely give to dogs of all sizes can be up to ten times the potency required to challenge the immune system of a Great Dane. She gave me two explanations for why this happens, despite that it makes little sense and is unsafe.

One explanation is that, in the field of immunology, overkill is thought to be beneficial. So, if for example you stimulate the immune system against distemper three times and you get the outcome you seek, then stimulating the immune system ten times is even better.

The other explanation has to do with receptor sites in the immune system for the particles that are being put into the bloodstream with the vaccines. The heavier the individual, the more receptor sites. So, to be safe, if you put way more particles into the body, you're making sure that proper immune stimulation is accomplished. Never once was there a proper explanation to what happens with all those other foreign viral and other introduced materials for which there are no longer any receptor sites, and which are immune challenging and harmful.

When I had my *Ask Martha's Vet* radio show on SiriusXM, I invited Dr. Ron Schultz to talk about vaccines and vaccine potency. Dr. Schultz—introduced earlier in this chapter—is a professor and former chair of the Department of Pathobiological Sciences at the University of Wisconsin–Madison School of Veterinary Medicine. He's the veterinarian who was doing all the research on vaccine immunity at the School of Veterinary Medicine and was working hand in hand with Dr. Dodds for many years. During the show, I asked, "Dr. Schultz, is it true that the potency of the vaccine could be up to ten times what the Great Dane needs?"

"Yes."

"Could you share with the listening audience why that is?"

That was a loaded question—I expected that Dr. Schultz would repeat one of the two reasons offered by Dr. Dodds.

"Shelf life," he replied. "They make the vaccine ten times stronger than its required potency so it'll last longer in the veterinarian's refrigerator."

To which I responded, live on the air, "Oh my God. So, is it a crapshoot, depending on when the veterinarian bought the vaccine?"

"Unfortunately, yes."

Welcome to science applied to health care!

The next day, I called Dr. Dodds and told her what Dr. Schultz had said on air, as the two had been such close associates for years. She said, "Why didn't Ron ever tell me that?"

FORCE OF HABIT

I hope that one day the veterinary profession will wake up to the routine overvaccination of the dogs and cats in our care—we're introducing powerful agents into their bodies when in many cases they simply don't need them. They already have all the immunity they need from previous rounds of vaccinations, and this has been shown through scientific verification.

To achieve this change, one of the first things that has to be overcome is the disbelief that something might be wrong with the way we vaccinate. I've heard that thousands of times. I'll be talking with a pet parent about their animal companion's vaccination schedule, and most of them are in disbelief that I'm even discussing this because it's such an accepted thing.

Someone will bring his or her dog in for some chronic illness or when the dog is not responding to conventional therapy. The first thing I ask as I go through the history is "How is she on her vaccinations?"

People will proudly reply, "She's up-to-date on all her vaccines!"

When I start to challenge that concept and get a blank stare, I ask, "When was your last polio shot?"

They'll always respond to that question with a chuckle.

"Oh, are *you* up-to-date on all *your* vaccinations?" I'll ask. That's when they get it.

"So, why are they different than us?" I'll continue. "It's scientifically proven that they're not."

In 2006, Dr. Ron Schultz published a comprehensive and

in-depth study of the duration of immunity for canine and feline vaccines.[7] Check out the minimum duration of immunity (DOI) for some common dog and cat vaccinations, according to Dr. Schultz's paper:

VACCINE	MINIMUM DOI	METHODS USED TO DETERMINE
CANINE DISTEMPER VIRUS (CDV) ROCKBORN STRAIN	7 YRS/15 YRS	CHALLENGE/SEROLOGY
CANINE DISTEMPER VIRUS (CDV) ONDERSTEPOORT STRAIN	5 YRS/9 YRS	CHALLENGE/SEROLOGY
CANINE ADENOVIRUS-2 (CAV-2)	7 YRS/9 YRS	CHALLENGE-CAV-1/SEROLOGY
CANINE PARVOVIRUS-2 (CPV-2)	7 YRS/9 YRS	CHALLENGE/SEROLOGY
CANINE RABIES	3 YRS/7 YRS	CHALLENGE/SEROLOGY

The following charts—created by Dr. Jean Dodds—are useful vaccine protocols for minimal vaccine use in dogs and cats:

Canine vaccine protocol

Note: The following vaccine protocol is offered for those dogs where minimal vaccinations are advisable or desirable. Dr. Dodds recommends this schedule, and it should not be interpreted to mean that other protocols recommended by a veterinarian would be less satisfactory. It's a matter of professional judgment and choice.

AGE OF PUPS	VACCINE TYPE
9–10 WEEKS	DISTEMPER + PARVOVIRUS, MLV (E.G. INTERVET PROGARD PUPPY DPV, *RENAMED NOBIVAC DPV* WHEN MERCK AND INTERVET MERGED)
14 WEEKS	SAME AS ABOVE
18 WEEKS	SINGLE MONOVALENT PARVO VACCINE *ONLY* (E.G. NEOPAR)
20 WEEKS OR OLDER, IF ALLOWABLE BY LAW	RABIES
1 YEAR	DISTEMPER + PARVOVIRUS, MLV (*OPTIONAL* = TITER)
1 YEAR *AFTER THE INITIAL DOSE*	RABIES, KILLED 3-YEAR PRODUCT (USE A THIMEROSAL [MERCURY]-FREE VACCINE, AND GIVE 3-4 WEEKS *APART* FROM DISTEMPER/PARVOVIRUS BOOSTER)

Perform vaccine antibody titers for distemper and parvovirus every three years thereafter, or more often if desired. Vaccinate for rabies virus according to the law, except where circumstances indicate that a written waiver needs to be obtained from the primary care veterinarian. In that case, a rabies antibody titer can also be performed to accompany the waiver request. See www.rabieschallengefund.org.

Feline vaccine protocol

Note: The following vaccine protocol is offered for those cats where minimal vaccinations are advisable or desirable. Dr. Dodds recommends this schedule, and it should not be interpreted to mean that other protocols recommended by a veterinarian would be less satisfactory. It's a matter of professional judgment and choice.

AGE OF KITTENS	VACCINE TYPE
8–9 WEEKS	RHINOPNEUMONITIS, CALICIVIRUS, PANLEUKOPENIA VIRUS (FVRCP)
12–13 WEEKS	SAME AS ABOVE
24 WEEKS OR OLDER, IF REQUIRED BY LAW	RABIES (E.G. MERIAL PUREVAX, RECOMBINANT)
1 YEAR	FVRCP BOOSTER
1 YEAR AFTER THE INITIAL DOSE	RABIES, SAME AS ABOVE BUT SEPARATED BY 2–3 WEEKS FROM FVRCP

Perform vaccine antibody titers for panleukopenia virus every three years thereafter, or more often if desired. Vaccinate for rabies virus according to the law, except where circumstances indicate that a written waiver needs to be obtained from the primary care veterinarian. In that case, a rabies antibody titer can also be performed to accompany the waiver request. See www.rabieschallengefund.org.

When I was a second-year vet student at Cornell, I lived on the outskirts of Ithaca in a nice apartment complex. On the top tier—two stories above me—lived a new resident at the veterinary college, Dr. Fred Scott. Nice guy! He went on to become probably the most notable veterinary virologist in the history of Cornell. Years back, he conducted a study on litters of cats standardly vaccinated up to one year of age for feline distemper (officially, *panleukopenia*). These litters were then challenged yearly with live viruses for this disease.

The results showed that immunity lasted a minimum of seven years, and sometimes a lifetime. This study was published in *JAVMA* (the *Journal of the American Veterinary Medical Association*).

The Rabies Challenge Fund (RCF) is scientifically demonstrating that the minimal length of protection generated by proper rabies immunization in dogs up to or a little older than one is five years. While the RCF study was originally to extend to seven years, the virus required to continue the study was not available from the USDA. Further, the rabies virus antibody titers of the study beagles fell below what is considered acceptable after about six and a half years. The formal paper from this research appears in the April 2020 issue of the *Canadian Journal of Veterinary Research*.

So, with these scientific studies mentioned above, why for decades were we vaccinating pets *every* year? Force of habit, and certainly not science. Thankfully, Dr. Jean Dodds, at the International Symposium on Animal Vaccines in 1997, got the recommendations changed to every three years.

But if studies are showing five-, seven-, nine-year—even lifetime—duration, why aren't we going there? We recently had a small dog in our clinic with cancer. While going through the patient's history, we came upon this statement:

The rabies vaccination your pet has just received has been medically tested to be effective for a period of 3 years. However, because of the epidemic propor-

tion of rabies occurring in this area, we strongly recommend that your pet be revaccinated on an annual
basis.

In researching the reported incidence of all rabid animals
in that area, I found it to be a grand total of two rabid rac-
coons in that year. Talk about a marketing ploy! Talk about
violating the Hippocratic oath to do no harm!

So, how should pets be properly vaccinated? This should
always be discussed and worked out on an individual doctor-
client-patient basis and not just with blanket recommendations. And, please, seek out a veterinarian who is well
educated on this subject and not governed by old habits or
standards. I tend to adhere to Dr. Dodds's charts above.

One more thing: On the package insert for every dog
or cat vaccine, a warning typically says something along
the lines of "Vaccinate healthy animals only." I can't even
count how many animals I've seen with a disease that got
vaccinated—because the calendar said it was time. Or even
worse, the law mandates it. And that's just in the case of
veterinary offices. Imagine how many sick animals get vaccinated each year—for little or no money—in large-scale
vaccination clinics, such as the ones offered by big-box pet
stores, humane societies, and dog and cat rescues.

If you look at the number of seconds in a year, and the
number of registered dogs and cats in the United States, doing the math, I come up with a conservative estimate that
1.5 dogs or cats get vaccinated every second if pets are vaccinated every three years. If vaccinated every year, the rate
just increases.

As Dr. Schultz explains, vaccination is ultimately a medical decision that should entail the same considerations and reasoning skills required when selecting an appropriate medical treatment or a specific surgical procedure. I ask you as a conscientious and loving pet parent to gently challenge your veterinarians on this topic. Explain your concerns and show them Dr. Dodds's vaccine protocols for minimal vaccination. Have them explain to you why your animal companions need to be vaccinated and on what schedule. If you're not satisfied with their response, then consider your options before you proceed.

Don't let your animal companions become victims of habit!

SOFIE'S STORY

When Sofie was first brought to Smith Ridge, she was a three-year-old, eleven-pound dog. You couldn't even tell her breed because of the disease that was eating through a good part of her nose. When you looked at her, she had the classical clinical signs of severe autoimmune disease—either discoid lupus or pemphigus, but it was also possibly a swarming cancer. (Keep in mind how we previously discussed the tie between autoimmune disease and vaccinations in the allergic breakthrough phenomenon.)

As we reviewed her medical history, we learned that Sofie was initially taken to a veterinarian on February 6. Although she had this severe condition, she was given vaccinations for seven different disease components at the same time because she was a stray. Where in nature does any individual have its immune system challenged by seven different diseases at the same time *by injection*, which bypasses nature's routes of protection?

On February 21, Sofie went back in. The disease on her face had significantly progressed—it was literally eating away her nose and her cheek. She was sedated for a sample for diagnosis. While under sedation, Sofie received vaccinations for seven more diseases. Although my associates and I have over the decades seen countless incidents like this with chronically sick pets, this is I think one of the highest levels of malpractice I've ever seen.

She was brought to us in this sad state. Her entire body was being eaten by this disease, and her back had welts and sores all over. This, to me, is attempted murder. It so violates the Hippocratic oath that we doctors swear to uphold. I'm sure that the veterinarian who initially treated Sofie is caring and just needs a wake-up call like the rest of those of our profession. The problem lies deeper, in the educational system, which is not willing to put proper science and studies into the efficacy, adverse effects, and duration of immunity of vaccinations.

The good news is that, after we treated Sofie, she dramatically improved and is now living a happier life, and her severely diseased areas are healing.

The other insanity is how we mandate animals to get vaccines before being boarded or going to a dog show or on an airplane. When people ask me about that, I just look at them and ask, "Have you ever gone to a Broadway play or a movie? Or stayed in a hotel?"

"Of course," they'll respond.

"Did you get vaccinated before you went?"

And they get it.

Why do our animal companions have to be vaccinated so often when we humans do not? I'll let you in on a little secret: they don't. Be as conscientious about your animal companions' vaccination schedules as you are about the food you feed them, the veterinarian you choose to keep them healthy, and the people in whose care you put them. Work closely with your veterinarian to adopt a minimal vaccination schedule, according to where you live, that protects your animal companions while not exposing them to unnecessary risks.

As cherished members of our family, they deserve at least this much from us, if not far more.

I would like to give a sincere thanks to my "sister in crime," Dr. Jean Dodds, for her excellent contributions to the contents of this chapter.[8]

ASK DR. MARTY

Q: I am concerned with having to get my two little poodles vaccinated and would like to put them on a minimal vaccination schedule, but my groomer and dog-boarding facility require that I provide proof that all vaccinations are up-to-date. What can I do?

A: This question has been bothering me ever since I realized that not only are adverse reactions associated with vaccinations, but that the immunity generated by them far exceeds what we have traditionally believed or accepted. Giving vaccinations on a fixed schedule—every year or two or three—has become such an accepted idea and practice that most people I meet just assume it's the right thing to do.

I am not anti-vaccine. But I am against how we have come to accept standardization practices for our companion animals and am dedicating a big part of my professional career to educate and do something about it.

In my experience, different groomers have different vaccination requirements. I suggest you shop around or consider using a mobile groomer who comes to your home, where no other dogs will be present. In the case of boarding your poodles, my best recommendation is don't do it. Instead, get a reliable pet sitter or relative to care for your animal companions—in your home or theirs. If you must board, then look for facilities that accept a minimal vaccination schedule. Many are now accepting titers for distemper and parvo showing proof of immunity (see the above section on titers for more information about that). You can do an internet search for minimal-vaccination boarding facilities in your area or check with your veterinarian. In addition, if your animal companion has a history of chronic illness, you can try to get a medical exemption.

As I write this book, we are in the midst of one of the worst global situations I have experienced in my lifetime: the COVID-19 global pandemic. I hope that by the time you are reading this, it has become history.

My concern, with reference to this chapter, is that companies are frantically trying to create vaccines to address the disease and are under considerable pressure to push them into society with only limited postvaccinal study. In a White House Coronavirus Task Force press briefing on March 26, 2020, Dr. Anthony Fauci described the potential risks to this hasty approach:

> Now, the issue of safety—something that I want to make sure the American public understand[s]: It's not only safety when you inject somebody and they get maybe an idiosyncratic reaction, they get a little allergic reaction, they get pain. There's safety associated—"Does the vaccine make you worse?" And there are diseases in which you vaccinate someone, they get infected with what you're trying to protect them with, and you actually enhance the infection.[9]

As I have seen over my decades of vaccine research, these epidemic diseases eventually tend to self-limit, especially globally. By the time they do, however, the vaccine is out there with government-mandated administration, and people—out of fear of the disease, often hyped by media—are themselves by the millions demanding to get the vaccine. Not only is this going to disrupt natural herd health going forward, as we have already discussed, but what adverse reactions and deep-seated health issues will result?

Perhaps by the time you read these words, we'll all know the answer to those questions.

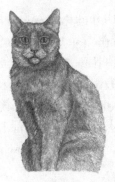

9

WALKING THROUGH YOUR PET'S SPIRITUAL WORLD

I think dogs are the most amazing creatures; they give
unconditional love.
For me, they are the role model for being alive.
—GILDA RADNER

Before we get into the heart of this chapter, I think it would
be good to take a minute to reflect on the sheer enormity
of this universe we live in with our animal companions.
Says Neil deGrasse Tyson, astrophysicist and director of the
Hayden Planetarium:

There are more stars in the universe than grains of
sand on any beach, more stars than seconds have
passed since Earth formed, more stars than words
and sounds ever uttered by all the humans who ever
lived.[1]

And I would posit that the amount of love on our planet Earth far outweighs the total mass of all those stars.

On the eve before New Year's Eve, I took my family out for Chinese food. At the end of the meal, we all cracked open our fortune cookies—looking forward to whatever inspiring messages awaited us. I opened my cookie and was surprised by just how profound my own fortune was:

Love in its essence is spiritual fire.

We humans have all sorts of characteristics that make us who we are. We're pretty smart, we have figured out how to use tools, we create art, we sing and make music. But one thing, I think, makes us truly human (or at least *should*):

Love.

Similarly, our dog and cat companions have all sorts of characteristics that make them who *they* are. They're pretty smart, they have great visual acuity, their olfactory capabilities are off the charts, they're loyal, and so on. However, like people, one thing makes dogs and cats what *they* truly are:

Love.

And with them, there is no *should*.

Love is the spiritual fire that we all share, and that we give abundantly and freely to one another. I believe the power of love allows us to transcend our usual earthly tethers and connections, and to commune with one another on a spiritual level. Every member of the animal kingdom—humans, whales, monkeys, pigs, chickens, dogs, cats, and on and on—joined together on a transcendent spiritual plane.

Powered by love.

The love we share with our animal companions.

Clive Wynne is a psychologist and founder of the Canine Science Collaboratory at Arizona State University and author of the book *Dog Is Love*. According to Wynne, what makes dogs particularly remarkable is not their intelligence. Instead, it's their ability to build affectionate relationships with one another, and with other species of animals.

They have the ability to love.

In a *Washington Post* interview, Wynne explains,

> I'm on record as one of the vehemently anti-anthropomorphic animal behavior scientists. Anthropomorphism means ascribing human qualities to animals. And certainly love is something we know first through human experience. But I think that different species can have different forms of love.
>
> Dogs fall in love much more easily than people do, and they also seem to be able to move on much more easily than people can. A lot of people have anxiety about the idea of adopting an adult dog. Wouldn't the dog be pining for its original human family? But what evidence we have indicates that dogs can form new loving relationships much more easily and don't seem to have the same level of trauma from being taken away from preexisting loving relationships.
>
> I'm not saying human and dog love are identical. I'm just saying there's enough similarity between how dogs form strong emotional bonds and how people form strong emotional bonds that it's fair enough to use the love word.[2]

I'm convinced that we humans and our animal companions share a bond so deep and profound that we are able to communicate with each other—from just a few feet away, to thousands of miles. We share biochemical and electromagnetic links that have been forged over millennia of mutual coexistence, friendship, and love. Here's a story that brings it all home. First, please fasten your grasp-of-reality seat belts.

Some years ago, when I had my weekly SiriusXM satellite-radio show on the Martha Stewart Living channel, an amazing animal communicator, Sonya Fitzpatrick, also had her own show on a neighboring SiriusXM channel, and I was asked by my producer Jocelyn to invite her on my show as a guest. She blew me away with some of the things she told the people calling in from all across the country about their pets.

During this time, my family made a major move from a New York home across the border about ten miles into Connecticut. You can imagine how crazy it was—three young daughters, all our furniture, a million boxes, and lots of animal companions. It was insane!

One of our two cats was Squeeki. My wife, when she was getting her tires changed at a local automobile repair shop, had found the cat in a cigarette bucket. The tiny kitten was only days old—she looked like a cross between a mouse and a baby bird. Someone—either human or cat mama—must have abandoned her. My wife brought the kitten home in her pocket. We nursed it back to health, and she became the most regal, elegant, Egyptian-looking cat you've ever seen.

A few days after we moved into our new home, while we were trying to add some order to the intense disorder, we lost track of Squeeki. She had somehow gotten out of the house and gone who knew where. After we'd searched for hours everywhere, Squeeki was nowhere to be found. She would squeak at you if she heard her name called, but no squeaks to be heard—no Squeeki.

We were freaked-out. We lived on a private road at the end of a cul-de-sac. As you drove up the road, you went over a small hill. There were three houses there, then two more houses on the private drive heading out to the main road. We went over to one of the homes directly across from us and introduced ourselves to one of the teens who lived there— sixteen-year-old John. We asked, "We lost our cat—have you seen one around here?"

"No, but there are a lot of coyotes around here."

Thank you, John.

We had heard these stories about cats finding their way back home, many miles away. So, we were now thinking, "Oh my God—we moved ten miles away, through the woods from New York to Connecticut, is she trying to find her way back home?"

On my second or third day of searching—while the rest of my family was driving the neighborhood—I went out the back door of our new home, made a left turn, and walked into the woods behind three more houses all the way down the block. Still no Squeeki. Frustrated and worried, I returned home. Then it hit me—I listed a bunch of animal communicators in my first book. Maybe one of them could help us. Or, even better, what about the animal communicator I had had on my radio show a few months earlier?

But for the life of me, I couldn't remember her name.

Suddenly, the new BlackBerry phone I rarely used vibrated

as I approached our house. I looked at it, and the first thing I saw was a Gillette razor ad. Scrolling down, I saw that the third message was from my SiriusXM show producer, Jocelyn. In the subject line of the email to me was the name Sonya Fitzpatrick—the animal communicator whose name I was trying so hard to remember. Coincidence?

Sonya was born with a hearing loss, and she found it easier to communicate with animals than with humans as she was growing up. That's what helped return her to hearing. The text of the email said, "Sonya would like to reciprocate and have you as a guest on her show. Are you interested?"

I called Joslin immediately. I asked her to call Sonya and tell her that I was absolutely interested, but I needed her to do me a huge favor. I'd lost my cat. Could she help me?

Within just a few minutes, I got a call from Sonya: "I don't really do this, but because it's you, I will try."

After a few moments of silence, Sonya began to talk: "Squeeki is still with us. She went out of your house to the left." This made me initially doubt Sonya—I had already gone out of the house that way and called and called for Squeeki, and I know she would have responded to me.

Sonya continued, "She's pretty close by. She is very freaked-out by a new noise she's hearing and it's scaring her." We now lived about a mile from a small airport, and planes were going over all the time. "I'm seeing a black Lab and a white trellis."

"A black Lab?" I handed the phone to my wife, and she told Sonya that the neighbor across the way—the one whose son had told us about the local coyote population—had a black standard poodle. My wife asked Sonya, "Do you mean a black standard poodle?"

"No. I see a black Lab and a white trellis."

So, we're starting to think that this lady is crazy, or at least downright wrong.

Then she said, "One way you could help find her is to collect your own urine and sprinkle it around."

That was about enough. We thanked Sonya for her information and said goodbye. My wife and I looked at each other and both said at the same time, "That was pretty useless." But it *was* a little comforting having her say that Squeeki was still with us.

The next day was Thursday, my day off, and Arnold and Karen—our neighbors down the road—invited us over to welcome us into the neighborhood. To get to their little house in the woods, we walked out our front door and turned to the left. Yikes—out the house to the left. I never considered the *front* door. As we made our way up the private drive to their house, we saw a white trellis. And there—sitting on the front porch—was a three-and-a-half-foot statue of a black Labrador retriever, a gift given to them in memory of their black Lab who'd passed.

We freaked out.

Instead of knocking on the door, we walked around the house because Sonya told us that she had seen this same view through Squeeki's eyes. We called out, "Squeeki, Squeeki, Squeeki!"

Nothing happened.

So, we all went into Arnold's house. We had some hors

d'oeuvres and tea, and our youngest daughter began to feel ill. My wife took her home, and sitting on our back porch was Squeeki. Sonya lived in Houston, Texas, and we lived in Connecticut—how the hell did she see this? If you stop for a few seconds and think about this—instead of just saying, "That's amazing!"—it changes your entire concept of reality.

After that, I had Sonya as a guest on my show three or four times more. People would call in and ask her questions. One call was from Canada about a dog with a behavioral issue. Sonya said to the lady, live on the air, "By the way, she wants you to know that she really likes the little blue bones painted on the bottom of her new water bowl."

The caller from Canada freaked out a bit. "How do you know that?"

Sonya continued to advise her, and then we were ready to hang up the call. In her British accent, Sonya told the caller, "Oh, by the way, darling, your orange cat sitting on the chair in the kitchen just wants you to know that it *was* a bladder problem."

The lady went ballistic with disbelief, and I didn't know how to respond. This was going out live, across the United States and Canada, to thousands of people. The only thing I could think of to say was "Sonya, how much did you pay this lady to call in today?"

Let's look at our universe from an electromagnetic perspective—not just using the five senses we have all been taught about since we were children. Sonya was somehow able to perceive Squeeki's thoughts and visions. When you leave physical consciousness, then all of a sudden there are no boundaries. That Sonya was in Houston, and I was more than fifteen hundred miles away, and a listener was in eastern Canada, didn't make a difference. Light travels at the speed of light. How fast does thought travel? If thought is an electromagnetic phenomenon, then it could travel at the same speed as light. And at 186,282 miles per second, that's pretty fast.

Think about the spirit of play that animals have, and how that affects the human race. They connect to art and music; you can stream music or play CDs that will help animals heal. I've had dogs who'd had their leg amputated, and the next day they're out in the field next to our hospital playing Frisbee. Amputate a person's leg, and they're in psychotherapy for months or years. Dogs and cats don't carry the mental baggage we humans do.

One thing we see time and time again is that disease in companion animals increases around holidays, especially Christmas and New Year's. It's not because, all of a sudden, we have poisonous plants such as poinsettias sitting around for our dog and cat companions to eat. It's because of all the stress and craziness that we humans go through. It changes the energetics of the environment globally and affects animals.

Is it any coincidence that dogs, and especially cats, somehow know the morning of their veterinarian's appointment and go hide in the closet? Or how they know that you're going on vacation? They'll just happen to get sick the day before. These are indicators of their ability to perceive something far more than through the five senses.

A good human cardiologist or MD will take your pulse on

your wrist and determine maybe two or three characteristics—the speed of the pulse, how strong it is, and the rhythm. A good acupuncturist can determine something like twenty-eight different characteristics. Something called the radial pulse is on the wrist, and all twelve paired acupuncture meridians have an energy on that pulse. So, the index finger, middle finger, and fourth finger—each picks up a different acupuncture meridian on that pulse. When light pressure is put on it, acupuncturists can pick up one set of six meridians, and with deep pressure, another. On top of all this, the speed and actual width of the pulse is factored into this diagnosis.

You'll go to see masters in acupuncture, and they will take your pulse for hours until they figure out what's going on. Then they could take maybe only one needle, stick it in one exact point, and you'll get better. It's because they know exactly what's going on, and they'll understand which of the 361 acupuncture points to target. A master will just do it—*boom*—like that. All these energetic things are far beyond the comprehension of classical medicine.

Then we have the MagnaWave. Several years ago, I lectured at their annual MagnaCon conference, and Dr. Amanda Myers—a pediatric emergency-medicine physician from Austin, Texas—also gave a lecture. Her partner—whose father is a veterinarian—had bought a MagnaWave machine. Dr. Myers said, "Ooh, I better study up on this unit that my partner bought, just to make sure that we're cool." She gave her lecture, and within the first eight minutes, I felt like giving her a standing ovation.

Why? Because she went to the chalkboard and explained in simple terms how and why this therapy works. Dr. Myers talked about how the physical body is in perfect balance with the earth. Remember the frequency of the earth from earlier in the book—the Schumann resonance at 7.83 Hz? This is the same energy we find in the human body when we look at the heart with an EKG and the brain with an EEG. Then Dr. Myers said:

What did we do? We paved the roads and highways. And what did we put on those highways? Tires made of rubber, which is an insulator. We wear shoes with rubber soles. We built buildings with metal reinforcement that insulate us from the earth. We use devices daily that create harmful energy. So, as we live with more exposure to harmful energy—and decrease our exposure to the healing earth energy—the physical body loses its energetic balance, leading to dysfunction and subsequently to disease. What the Magna-Wave does is, it reintroduces that energy into the body. This reestablishes proper energetic flows and it gets better.

And what is it that enables dogs to sense a seizure in a human companion before it starts? Or to sense the presence of disease? In one study, dogs were able to discern the blood samples from people who had cancer with an accuracy of 97 percent. Dogs have been found to know when humans are about to have a narcolepsy attack, or when a migraine is coming on, or when someone has low blood sugar, or when people are fearful or under stress. It may be linked to their remarkably powerful sense of smell, or maybe it's something more.[3] This just expands your electromagnetic consciousness of the physical universe and how they fit in with us and we fit in with them.

THE EXTRAPHYSICAL SENSES OF DOGS AND CATS

In addition to the many perceptions that we share with dogs and cats beyond those of the standard five senses—sight, hearing, smell, taste, and touch—our animal companions can do us one better. Some of their senses are far more powerful than the ones we humans have. For example, as mentioned earlier, dogs are able to sniff out lung cancer in humans with 97 percent accuracy.[4] And we all know that dogs can hear sound frequencies much higher than we can—the proverbial dog whistle. While humans can hear sounds only up to about 20,000 Hz, dogs are able to hear up to about 45,000 Hz. And cats are even higher—up to about 79,000 Hz.

In that sense, dogs and cats have perceptions that can be considered extraphysical—beyond what we humans can perceive. And not just when it comes to the traditional five senses, but some remarkable things as well. These extraphysical senses aren't magic, though sometimes they may seem that way. They are simply adaptations to the environments in which these animals live.

For example, whales and dolphins can navigate through the water—avoiding obstacles or locating prey—through echolocation, which is similar to the sonar systems used by boats and submarines. These animals send out a sound that bounces off another animal or object in the water and then echoes back—providing information on its size, location, and shape. And we all know the age-old adage "blind as a bat." How do they zoom around as fast as they do, know exactly where they are going, and catch their food with no problem? Echolocation. Although some people—especially blind individuals—have learned how to use echolocation, most people lack that ability.

Some dogs are born with the ability to sense oncoming seizures, minutes or even hours before they occur, in people with epilepsy. Recent research indicates that when a person is going to have a seizure, they emit a specific scent that some dogs can pick up on. Other research indicates that this ability may even have an electromagnetic component. Says Craig Angle, codirector of the Canine Performance Sciences Program in the College of Veterinary Medicine at Auburn University, "The dog is a natural biosensor, preprogrammed with thirty thousand years of evolutionary algorithms, and three hundred million sensory receptors." Dogs have been trained to sniff out bombs and track lost children (and escaped criminals). Some think they can smell fear—and even love.

Some animals are able to sense a coming hurricane and get out of the way. Sharks, for example, have been observed to move to deeper water before a hurricane, and birds may land on the ground and wait for the storm to go by before returning to the air. It's thought that the animals may detect a hurricane's low-frequency sound waves or that they are sensitive to changes in air or water pressure resulting from the coming storm.

When I studied acupuncture in 1975, I learned that storms and seasonal atmospheric changes create a tremendous amount of positively charged ions. As a *New York Times* article explained, these weather conditions—and the ions that are generated—have the power to "affect people's mood and health, even precipitating suicides, crimes, and accidents."[5] If they have such a great impact on us humans, imagine the impact these positive ions have on our animal companions!

Although it is unproven, many emergency medical personnel have long believed that a full moon and increased emergency room visits, childbirths, bleeding, and more are directly correlated.[6] As I always say, if the moon can trigger tides that raise the ocean level by three feet or more, imagine what it could do to the pressures in your body and in your head—especially when you consider that up to 60 percent of the adult human body is composed of water and the brain is 73 percent water.[7] Where do you think the term *LUNAtic* comes from?

Bees can sense the earth's magnetic field, and platypuses and sharks can tune in to the electrical impulses of prey—accurately locating them. Some species of snakes can see in the dark by detecting the infrared radiation given off by animals and objects, sea turtles can sense the earth's magnetic field and navigate using it, and jewel beetles can detect the presence of fire (a burning pine tree) up to ten miles away.

Cats gained prominence in ancient Egypt, where they were associated with different gods and deities. According to Smithsonian Institution curatorial fellow Antonietta Catanzariti, "Everything had a meaning. A cat protecting the house from mice. Or it might just protect kittens. Those were attitudes that were attributed to a specific goddess."[8] For example, an image of Bastet—the goddess of motherhood—in the form of a cat was found carved into a column. Lions represented royalty. It's no wonder why the ancient Egyptians elevated cats in their culture.

Melinda Hartwig, curator of ancient Egyptian, Nubian, and Near Eastern art at Emory University's Michael C. Carlos Museum in Atlanta, emphasizes, however, that those early Egyptians did not actually worship cats—they did not consider them to be gods or goddesses. Instead, cats were believed to contain the divine spirit of Bastet. When the cult of Bastet was at its pinnacle in the second century BCE, cat charms and amulets were commonly worn by people for good luck and protection, and mummified cats were all the rage. Says Hartwig, "Mummified cats would be sold to pilgrims who would go to the temple of the goddess Bastet and give the goddess back a little bit of her energy. They would also ask for a favor in the form of a prayer, known as a votive."

Fast-forward to today. You'll be looking at a cat just sitting relaxed on the other side of the room, then, all of a sudden, its tail will flick back and forth, and its ears will start to jump and flutter. Is the cat detecting incoming extraphysical energies—something you can't detect with your own five senses? I once learned in a seminar way back in the seventies that this is exactly the role of cats for us humans—to serve as detectors of incoming energies for us. And all that flicking is their way of balancing the energies being thrown at us.

Perhaps. No one knows for sure.

ASK DR. MARTY

Q: I've heard it said that animals are nowhere near as spiritually advanced as we humans are. Working with them as long as you have, what is your opinion about that?

A: I couldn't disagree more! Consider the words of novelist and playwright Frances Hodgson Burnett in her 1905 book, *A Little Princess:*

> *How it is that animals understand things I do not know, but it is certain that they do understand. Perhaps there is a language which is not made of words and everything in the world understands it. Perhaps there is a soul hidden in everything and it can always speak, without even making a sound, to another soul.*

How does a dog know its guardian is going to have a seizure hours before it comes on? How do animals know a tsunami is coming and migrate upland to safety when man has no idea that disaster is imminent? How does your dog know you are leaving work many miles away? Intelligence does not necessarily equate to spirituality. We have many lessons to learn from animals. All we need to do is open ourselves to doing just that.

One of the interesting things about my having a high profile in the world of veterinary medicine is that I often receive emails, notes, and letters from pet parents who want to tell me their amazing stories. And believe me, I have received some amazing stories in addition to the ones I've personally collected in more than forty-five years of clinical practice! Here's one from Kelli Swan, which arrived while I was writing this book. Let it serve as an example of the many more I could share:

> I wanted to share how thoroughly blown away I was with *The Dog Doc*, and your book. I've been living an integrative lifestyle for decades, and trying to do that with my dogs. Your information is helping me take both to a whole new level. I also purchased *Emmanuel's Book*, which echoes the teachings of so many others (*Conversations with God*, Eckhart Tolle, Abraham Hicks, etc.). Both books are now my handy references.
>
> After reading the chapter in your book, I had a bit of an epiphany. I'd like to share it with you. :-)
>
> In your chapter on The Spiritual Realm, you shared some of the many cases where pets were mirroring their owners' illnesses. I've experienced the same thing on many occasions with my pets. One case was a stunner.
>
> At the time, I was dealing with a rather dysfunctional personal relationship. During a phone conversation, my boyfriend at the time shared something so hurtful that I broke down sobbing. The conversation was just one of many unpleasant ones, and I had reached my breaking point. I cried so hard that my chest actually hurt. About a week later, my dear dog Sunny came down with sudden onset DCM [canine dilated cardiomyopathy]. She died a week after that. One of my spiritually inclined friends said, "She took on your heartache for you."

I never forgot that thought—it brings tears to my eyes to this day. As Emmanuel says, all disease manifests first in the nonphysical plane. I heard another spiritual teacher (can't remember which one now) say that the "beasts of our world" are here to counterbalance human negativity, so we can better learn our lessons and evolve. The animals are actually part of us and came here for that very role.

My epiphany is this: The increasing amount of cancers and other ailments we see in our pets are not just due to food, vaccines, toxins, etc. Our pets are "taking on our fears" so that we may evolve. They are helping us, much as one would use a walker or cane. As Emmanuel says, cancer is fear made manifest, and we humans are certainly experiencing no small amount of fear as we learn. :-)

I've gotten to the point that if one of my dogs has a health issue, I do an internal inventory of what's going on in my life, and how I'm reacting to it. It's been revealing, to say the least.

Twenty years ago, I made the acquaintance, by telephone, of Dr. Rick Palmquist, a practicing veterinarian on the outskirts of Los Angeles. I had heard of him and he of me. However, the news about me was quite alarming to him because, hearing from one of his clients that consulted with me that I was approaching cancer using diet and supplements, truly rubbed him the wrong way. He was on a secret mission to get my license suspended. Pretending to be interested in my work in the phone conversation, he asked how he could learn about this. Jokingly, I said I was giving a long seminar on the subject at the end of the week in Connecticut. He said, "I'll be there." I picked him up at LaGuardia, he came to my five-hour Kodachrome slide presentation, spent two days at my clinic, reviewing records, meeting patients and clients, and his life was changed forever. Weeks later he actually told me that what he experienced was so powerful, so deep within him, that he went to his ophthalmologist a week later to get his eyes examined and his vision and eyeglass prescription actually improved. He subsequently became a column writer on integrative veterinary medicine for *The Huffington Post* and after serving as president of the American Holistic Veterinary Medical Association, he headed the research committee for the American Holistic Veterinary Medical Foundation (a charitable organization that everyone reading this book should donate to).

Here is my friend and colleague, Dr. Rick Palmquist:

THE ESSENCE OF ANIMAL HEALING

BY RICHARD E. PALMQUIST, DVM, GDVCHM, ACCHVM

Centinela Animal Hospital, Inc.

The nature of animal healing is this pure essence of survival. Animals don't complicate their lives with lies and politics. They breathe in, take what they need, then exhale the waste and move on.

People worry about breathing.

Animals just breathe.

And when they are sick, they go somewhere safe to rest, fast, and recover. It's what they do. And if we watch, listen, and learn from them, it's what we should do as well.

Timer was an old dog I'd been helping for a long time. Working with internal medicine specialists, our health team helped him survive aging, arthritis, diabetes, and Cushing's disease (a small brain tumor making his body produce too much cortisone). After recovering in ICU from a severe stroke, he went home. A few days later, his guardian called to report a sudden fall and pain after going downstairs. Timer came to the office and X-rays revealed severe bone cancer and a pathological fracture. The cancer had eaten away the bone until it was so weak it simply broke.

This was devastating news. I explained the facts to Timer's mother, Karen. It seemed euthanasia was appropriate, but Karen simply said, "No, not today—do your magic. I'll take him home and we'll see."

Earlier in my career I would have been upset, but Dr. Marty taught me to try—to let the dog have a chance. He said, "Put in energy. See what the dog does with it. If he makes more of it, that's healing. Help it. If he just makes more cancer, you're done. Help him along his way."

So, we tried. In six weeks, Timer was walking. He still had cancer, but his bone healed and he lived a beautiful life for nearly a year. No chemo, no radiation, no surgery— only Love, a ton of prayer, a great diet, and supplements. Oh, and he made so many friends along the way.

What did Karen and Timer teach me?

The biggest lesson is simply the power and reality of Love as a force of universal creation and healing. The other was how Love connects, aligns, empowers, and creates our lives as a connected, vital activity.

Love is real.

The Chinese call it "good qi." They consider it to be a given in any healing effort.

Love connects all of Life from microorganisms to ecosystems. With Love, in Love—we are never alone; never without hope or genuine help.

If we love, life will connect us in wild ways to what we need. It connected me to Dr. Marty and changed my own health and the health of those around me.

Treatment is fiddling with parts, while healing is Love moving in ways that make Life better. And that is a group activity of a Greater Love being freed to work in our lives. That is a new culture transforming all it touches. It is the Source of Love manifesting its best expression of Love for this particular Now.

For me, that *is* the Spirit of Animal Healing as Love moves through our existence and awakens and connects us in better community. I loved Timer. Karen loved Timer. Together we found a way to free his desire to persist and enjoy his life.

That kind of Love set free becomes a new ethics, morality, law, and politics. It aligns our breath and our motion between soil, air, and water. It allows us to best use the resources we hold. It is an ecology and economics of stewardship favoring a larger sphere of improved mutual survival.

And it is the foundation of all meaningful education, as Love seeks truth, and shares it in ever-broader spheres.

Yes, Timer and Karen taught me that.

In its raw essence, that is what integrative medicine is all about. Love aligning nature and human understanding so spirit, mind, and body can connect and live better together.

Thank you for this, Rick. What you added here is at the highest level of true healing, *love*. And to be clear, we are talking about true love that is the highest level of admiration and devotion, and not the Hollywood variety of love that's no more than an entrapment.

CROSSING OVER—THE FINAL FRONTIER

Yes, we love our animal companions dearly, but eventually we all have to say goodbye—at least for *this* lifetime! Sometimes the departure from this world to the next happens in the blink of an eye, and sometimes it's a long, drawn-out process. No matter how the dogs and cats in our lives cross over, it's traumatic for all concerned.

We've all been through the pain of having to say our last goodbyes to a beloved animal companion—to look in her eyes one last time, to hold him in our lap as he takes his last breath, to bid a fond farewell. While this is a sad time, if your animal companion is extremely ill or has been suffering, then this can also be a time of great relief—even joy. Your dear friend won't have to suffer any longer and will feel no more pain. And as I discussed in my first book, you *can* be with him or her again—just in a different form.

When your dog or cat crosses over, do you want to be there? Will you be there? That's a question we all must face, and the right answer is that you should do whatever feels right for *you*.

I believe it might be better if you decide *not* to be in the room with your animal companion when he or she is euthanized. I received some vocal criticism from readers when I said this in my first book.

In nature, when animals are going to die, they know it's time. When it's time, they go off and do it on their own. It's *our* baggage that makes us feel we have to be there with them. Concerned pet parents will say to me, "Oh, no—I have to be there so she knows I love her." When my brother and I were veterinarians together, my brother had a Doberman named Emily. When it came time for her to pass, my brother's family all said their goodbyes to Emily and left their home. I was there with a technician and helped Emily cross. So, their memories were of Emily in life, not being euthanized.

I learned this lesson when I was a freshman at veterinary school. I had a young white cat who came down with feline leukemia. When she was euthanized at Cornell, I was in the room with her. Sadly, from that day onward, when I thought about her, the only thing I could see in my mind's eye was her being put to sleep.

So, I share these thoughts because it's an animal's great privilege in nature to go off on its own to die. Animals don't run to their family when it's time to go. I've had some pet parents who obsessed over this—that they had to be there when their animal companion was euthanized. Then, years later, when it was time for their next animal companion to cross over, I would suggest a different approach: They would say their goodbyes at home, especially with their children. Then they would have a neighbor or a family member drop off the dog or cat at Smith Ridge.

Afterward I would get a call along the lines of "Thank you so much because, when we think about our first pet, we think about her being euthanized. But with our second one, we only remember her in life."

If you want to be there during the final moments of your animal companion's life, I support you 100 percent. And with some of my own that have been helped to pass, I with my family have been there. So, please be there for them. But believe me, it's also 100 percent okay if you're not. On the nonphysical plane we just discussed, that *love* is felt.

Whether or not to euthanize can be one of the most difficult decisions you will ever make. Although I covered this in my first book, the topic is important enough to discuss again with advice from my experience.

To me, only one answer simplifies matters at such a difficult time: *you'll know when you know.*

Making this decision when you have a lot of doubt will tend to come back and haunt you. If someone asks me for my opinion, my answer is almost always "No, you're not ready. This is a lifelong relationship you, your family, and your pet have shared. Not your veterinarian. You will know when that balance tips beyond doubt to euthanasia."

As was so eloquently stated in *Emmanuel's Book II,*

"Euthanasia is merciful release from a body that no longer functions. In the center of your being, there is no doubt or confusion."[9] At that moment, I won't be asked for my opinion, but will be told, "It's time."

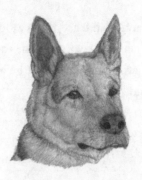

10

TAILS BEYOND THE CLINIC

There's always room for a story that can transport people
to another place.
—J. K. ROWLING

Over the decades, I have consulted for and treated thousands of dogs and cats. While I have become an accomplished veterinarian over the years, perhaps my number-one skill outside of my veterinary practice is as a storyteller. You may have noticed that in the stories I've already told you.

While most of my encounters with dogs and cats were fairly routine and uneventful, some were remarkable and inspiring. In this chapter, you'll read some more of my most amazing, most remarkable stories, which I tell here for the first time.

O FOR OPRAH

Trust me. Although this is something to brag about and make my résumé look that much better, with all the other stories I've already shared, I would be remiss not to share this one. With her incredible love for animals, books, and hope that aligned closely with what my own life is about, making contact with Oprah was high on my radar. She had helped rocket the exposure and success of Dr. Oz and others, and I had heard countless times from acquaintances that I was "the Dr. Oz of veterinary medicine." So, why not try to connect?

Before we did indeed meet each other, Smith Ridge was getting calls about ill pets every day from all across the country—many requesting my help ASAP. I never got on a phone call without people first going through a comprehensive protocol—registration forms, medical records sent, and a consultation appointment—usually weeks in advance.

One day, we received a call from Los Angeles from someone named Kate Forte about her cat, which had had part of his intestines removed and was not doing well. "Can you help?" she asked.

For some strange reason, and this is something I never do, when my receptionist asked if this was something we could help with, I told her, "Let me get on the phone."

Kate and I had a good talk, and I was about to have her set up a phone consult stat. I then asked her—as I do with most of my long-distance clients—if there was any way she could bring her animal companion to Smith Ridge. Kate responded that she was bicoastal and that it might be a possibility. When I heard this, just out of curiosity I asked her what she did, being bicoastal.

She explained, "I'm the president of Oprah's film company."

About thirty seconds later, after I picked myself up off the floor, I replied, "Oh, really?!"

As it turned out, Kate didn't need to fly in. I worked in coordination with her local veterinarian to continue proper medical therapy as I added in a comprehensive support program. Her cat made a full recovery.

Months later, Kate told me that Oprah had invited all the ladies who worked for her to a "girls' weekend retreat" at her mansion in Montecito, outside Santa Barbara. Then Kate said, "All I'm going to talk about, especially to O, is Dr. Marty."

Nothing happened for more than a year. One day, however, I was talking with Kate about her dog, and she said that O might be calling me about *her* dog.

Again, nothing came of it.

I had just gotten my own SiriusXM radio show by then, *Ask Martha's Vet*, and I had to commute one and a half hours by train into Manhattan, then hustle up to Forty-Eighth Street where the studios were housed.

I had just bought a new cell phone and hardly anyone had my number. I was supposed to call an 800 number to block advertising calls, but I forgot to do it. Just as the train was entering the tunnel that leads into Grand Central Station— which cuts cell phone service—I received a call from a number with more than ten digits. "Oh, great," I thought to myself, "it must be one of those advertising calls." When I left the station and walked out onto the street, my cell phone dinged—I had a voice-mail message. Thinking it was just an ad, I almost deleted it, but curiosity won out. I played the message.

"Hi, Dr. Marty, this is Oprah Winfrey calling. I'm calling you from South Africa. Kate Forte gave me your number. It's about my dog, Sophie. Please call me back at this number."

I couldn't make calls out of the United States with my new phone, so I called my wife, Meg, to ask her to call someone for me. It was right around dinnertime.

"Now?" she asked. "I'm feeding the kids—can't it wait? Who am I calling?"

"Oprah Winfrey. Just ask her to call me back."

Meg willingly agreed.

Oprah called me two more times, and the calls went direct to voice mail. The third time was the charm, and the call made it through to me. My phone rang and I immediately picked it up.

After Oprah said hello, I told her, "I have been anticipating this call for years, but never dreamed that when it came in, it would be from Africa to Grand Central Station!"

"Isn't technology wonderful?" marveled Oprah.

So, we discussed Sophie's condition, which I will not divulge other than to say a veterinarian recommended that Sophie get a surgical procedure to continue her therapy. Having doubts, Oprah wanted me to give her a second opinion. From what I was told and could ascertain about Sophie's condition, *my* recommendation was no. But, as we talked, I was approaching the SiriusXM studios and had minutes left to get on the air. I explained to Oprah that I would need to hang up. I guess not too many people say that to her! When she asked me why, I said that Martha Stewart had given me my own national radio show, and I was going on the air in just a few minutes.

"Oh, really!" Oprah replied.

After my show was over, Oprah and I picked up our conversation—further discussing the situation with Sophie. Oprah said, "I like what I'm hearing, so I will have her checked out of the hospital and flown to your clinic in the morning."

"No."

I could feel that Oprah was again taken aback.

When she asked me why not, I explained that you don't want to suddenly take a patient that has been hospitalized with her condition out of the hospital and onto a plane— even though it's yours and Sophie's accustomed to it—and ship her to another clinic that far away. The other thing I said is that I didn't want to be treating Oprah's dog when Oprah was that far away in Africa. We'd just be asking for trouble. Again, she agreed and told me that made sense. When she asked what she should do, I suggested she assign to me the person who typically cares for Sophie and I would work with her in Oprah's absence.

Enter Louise!

The next day, Tuesday, Sophie was discharged from the hospital and brought home. From the list Louise sent me, Sophie was on eleven different medications. Though not entirely surprised that she was on medications, I was a bit stunned by these many different things. I asked Louise, "What do you think would happen if you put a perfectly normal dog on all these medications?"

Louise smartly answered, "She'd probably get sick!"

Exactly! I was careful not to give direct medical advice, but I mentioned the three medications that I would have approved and maybe even used if Sophie were my in-house patient. Louise decided to cut out the other eight, and I had her start cooking "real" food for Sophie. By the time Friday came around, we were down to just one medication. Sophie was making great progress.

I got a call from Oprah on Saturday at 8:00 A.M. She said, "I landed back home hours ago, and when I walked in, Sophie did her Sophie dance for the first time in quite a while. I will be there Monday morning." This time I did *not* say no.

We canceled most of the appointments scheduled at the clinic at around Oprah's arrival time—noonish. A huge black SUV limo pulled into our parking lot, and several huge men walked into Smith Ridge with walkie-talkies in their wristwatches. Remember, this was 2007—way before the Apple watch! The coast was clear, and Oprah came into the waiting room dressed in all sweats, clutching Sophie as tightly as possible.

The pair were ushered into my exam room, and we spent about an hour together—typical for any new client. When discussing options, I explained the benefits of IV vitamin C therapy, which was indicated for Sophie. But Oprah said, "Before I leave Sophie here, I want a tour of the whole hospital." As we were wrapping up the tour of the clinic, she blurted out, "Damn, this place even *smells* good."

I immediately called the veterinarian I considered the

number one radiologist in the profession, Dr. Victor Rendano. He was the head technician in the radiology department at the Cornell veterinary school when I was a student there—he set up the radiology consulting service we used on our difficult cases. Besides being based just outside Ithaca, New York, where Cornell is, Victor would go out on the road as a traveling radiologist and certified ultrasonographer. I needed his input whether or not this was indeed an emergency surgical condition. But Dr. Rendano wasn't scheduled to be back until later in the week.

That wouldn't work.

However, when I mentioned whose dog we were talking about, Dr. Rendano immediately made the four- or five-hour drive to my clinic. He verified that this was indeed one of the more advanced cases of Sophie's condition that he had ever seen on sonogram. It wasn't a mandatory emergency surgery, but it could potentially worsen if not treated. I discussed all this with Oprah, and she decided that, considering Sophie's age, she preferred to avoid cutting her open.

So, for the rest of the week, we kept Sophie on a comprehensive IV vitamin C therapy program with great food we cooked for her and the introduction of specific supplements. She appeared to be doing well. Oprah sent a plane to pick Sophie up on Friday. The two met up at O'Hare Airport in Chicago and then flew to California.

That weekend I got an email from Oprah with some great news. She was in disbelief at how well Sophie was doing. That was music to my ears, and everything I'd hoped for.

After the weekend, Oprah and I spoke just before she was about to tape her show. As she shared her elation about how well Sophie was doing, I let her know that we still had a long way to go to establish stable healing. This is where I work hand in hand with local veterinarians. I informed her that this process works well, and that I never had any problems interacting with conventional veterinarians.

"But we have a problem here."

"What's the problem?" asked Oprah.

"Your veterinarian is Oprah Winfrey's vet!" There are some really big egos in the medical field, and I knew her current veterinarian wouldn't be happy to share Sophie's care with me, some *holistic* vet.

"You take care of Sophie," said Oprah. "I'll take care of my vet!"

She had to hang up and start her show. Her closing words were "I know, you had me at hello!"

When I heard those words, my heart almost stopped. We stayed in email contact. Days later, I heard from Oprah. She wanted to fly with Sophie to her home in Hawaii, but she had run up against a roadblock. Sophie couldn't fly to Hawaii without getting a rabies vaccine booster. That was the last thing Sophie needed given her medical history and age.

In the email to me, Oprah wrote, "Vets just don't get it!!"

We spoke shortly after—Oprah wanted to know if I had any advice. I didn't, but I jokingly asked, "Why don't you just buy the island?"

"Don't think I haven't thought about it!"

After that I had no more communications from Oprah, and no response to a few emails I sent her asking how Sophie was doing. This had me a bit concerned about Sophie's condition. Weeks later, on a Monday—just before noon—I was on a phone consultation with a good client who lived in the Midwest, not far from Chicago. My receptionist walked into my office and handed me a sticky note on which she'd written, "Oprah on line 2."

As I was about to ask my receptionist to get Oprah's number so I could call her back, I realized that probably wasn't wise. I told this to my consult, and he said, "Are you crazy? Take that call and call me back later."

I punched the button for line two and said, "Hello."

The first thing Oprah said to me was that she understood I was on the phone with someone from her area. How did she *know* that?

Then Oprah quickly said, "Have you heard from my people?"

I froze with fear. I hadn't heard from her in weeks. I figured Sophie's condition must have gotten really bad, and her vet blamed it all on me and my holistic, nonapproved treatments. I assumed when she said "my people," she was talking about her lawyers. I was watching my entire life go down the drain.

"I'm putting you on my show Wednesday," said Oprah, to my surprise and tremendous relief, "and I need you to fly to Chicago tomorrow."

There was just one problem: my wife, Meg, was planning a huge sixtieth birthday party for me, and it was to serve as a fundraiser for Dr. Jean Dodds and the Rabies Challenge Fund.

I stupidly replied to Oprah, "But I have this huge event on Saturday, and I haven't really done my share for it yet."

"Good, that gives you three days. I'll see you Wednesday." Oprah hung up.

The next day, I flew to Chicago. Oprah squeezed me into an already-planned show with her dog trainer, Tamar Geller. Oprah wanted me to talk about the big pet food recall. Even though I only had four and a half minutes on air, it was the experience of a lifetime—something I'll never forget.

At the end of the show, I was waiting for everyone else to start filing out. Instead, all the lights in the studio went dim. I had no idea what was happening. Suddenly, a spotlight went on Oprah, ready to start recording the Oprah after-show segment that streams to millions of people on her website.

Oprah started the segment by saying, "Okay, Dr. Goldstein, please tell them the truth about vaccinations."

I talked for more than a half hour, including a Q and A. I was ecstatic! I was finally going to get this vital message about vaccinations out to millions of people when it streamed a couple weeks later.

The day before the stream was to run, Oprah's producer called to tell me that, unfortunately, the legal department had cut it out. The good news is that I've been able to get out the truth about vaccinations in a variety of different ways, including the book you're now holding in your hands.

MAGGIE Q

Meet my adopted sister, so to speak, and adopted aunt to my three daughters. Years ago I was in the treatment area of my clinic when my associate Dr. Mike popped out of his exam room and said, "I've got this Hollywood-type chick in my room, and I think you and her would really hit it off. You should go meet her!"

So I went in, and as they say, the rest is history.

Maggie had just moved to our area from Los Angeles and was looking for a local veterinary facility to care for her three dogs. I was impressed by how much she knew about proper holistic care for them, and in what great shape they were for their ages and histories. Also, Maggie did look kinda familiar. She played Nikita on the TV series by the same name, but I never saw it. And, yes, she's the one who beat the crap out of Tom Cruise in the opening scene of *Mission Impossible 3*. We hit it off philosophically about life and health care and spent at least an hour talking.

And talk about an animal lover and supporter. Maggie is a big supporter of the David Sheldrick Wildlife Trust, which is on a quest to protect and save elephants with a focus on rescuing and rehabilitating orphaned infant elephants. I was impressed when I was invited to the Hollywood Palladium to attend PETA's thirty-fifth anniversary celebration, where Maggie received their Humanitarian of the Year award and Paul McCartney was the entertainment. During his performance, I was staring at Paul from eight feet away and was having a difficult time controlling my goose bumps.

And I'll never forget the day Maggie was on the set in Toronto filming for the series *Designated Survivor*, in which she costarred with Kiefer Sutherland, when the hurricane hit Houston. Maggie announced, "Hey, I gotta leave. I rented a plane and I'm flying down there to help rescue the animals." Yes, that's Maggie. I shared with her my excitement over my newfound therapy toy, my recently purchased Magna-Wave unit, and how blown away I was with the responses I was getting—not only in some of the dogs I treated with the unit, but also with some of my friends, employees, and myself.

Now on to Cesar, Maggie's regal German shepherd, which she adopted years back. Cesar was so together, so in tune, so intelligent, you'd swear that he was mostly human! He was in great shape on an exclusively raw diet that Maggie would prepare every day along with a bunch of good supplements. So, I just fine-tuned his program based on blood samples. All was great and he entered his teens. Suddenly, a small lump appeared under his skin in his rear abdomen. I took a sample of it by needle aspiration, and it revealed a common cancer called mast cell. I recommended no surgery and definitely no chemo. I just added in several more supplements I have specifically and successfully used for this cancer type and for allergies, since mast cells in the blood of normal dogs contain histamine.

Weeks later, Maggie contacted me to say, "Holy ____! It shrunk in half! Now, when I do any filming with you about this work, I no longer have to act!" Cesar did great for a couple more years and approached being a sixteen-year-old German shepherd still zipping around and enjoying life—something kinda rare these days. And with this I'd now like to introduce my adopted sister-in-crime, Maggie Q:

I was driving when I got the call from Marty. I remember I wasn't far from my house, and my vet and I are close friends who talk all the time, so it wasn't unusual to get a call from him. We did send out for a biopsy a few days earlier, but I'm the type of person who won't carry stress about something I don't know for certain. Animals pick up on everything we feel, and if you are as close to yours as I am to mine, there is no hiding. I remained positive for my boy, and he knew it.

I found the lump on him when I was filming in Atlanta. It didn't belong where it was, and it was definitely new. I told my dog that we would get it checked out and wouldn't worry about it until we had to. Even then, we would handle anything that came our way.

As life would have it, it did come our way. It's cancer, Marty told me.

My heart plummeted into my stomach, and I could feel my whole body seize up with fear. I immediately looked into my rearview mirror to check on Cesar. It was a severe energy shift for me, and I knew he would have picked up on it already.

As I pulled into my driveway and turned off the car, I reached for the release button on the car's back door. My boy knows not to jump out until he gets the okay, so I said it as enthusiastically as I could so he would go and roam the property and I could take a minute to absorb the conversation I just had. But today, he didn't. I said okay several more times as the door sat open and he wouldn't move.

It was clear to me that a conversation was needed, and he wasn't going anywhere until we had it.

Animals make you accountable in every moment. They are the purest form of instinct and generosity of spirit that I have ever known. I was upset, and my Cesar knew it. He wasn't going to let me gloss over it the way we humans do. Animals are too honest for that. If there was an issue, we were going to face it right there, together.

I took a deep breath, exited the driver's seat, and I climbed into the back of the car—unable to hide from my soul partner—and I cried. I told him I didn't even like if a tick hurt him, much less something more serious. I told him there was an issue with his health and that nothing was going to happen to him because I was going to do everything in my power to help him. I told him how strong he was, and how strong I was, and I meant every word of it.

Over the next several months, Marty and I had many discussions about what treatment would look like for Cesar. I knew that if I had had a different vet, it would have been by the book. Chemo or radiation, surgery, repeat. Pretty standard by Western veterinary methods, but that's not who I had looking after my boy and me. I had Marty, and I had Meg.

It's important to understand how these two changed the course of my animal's health, not only physically but also spiritually and psychologically. They empowered their own deep instincts, which in turn allowed me to trust mine. In that scary time, I found faith that rose above medicine—it was trust in the knowledge and, most of all, the animal itself.

Who trusts an animal to engage in its own healing? Marty does. One of my fondest memories of that time is Marty telling me, "We are going to do everything we can, the rest is up to him."

One of the most important phone calls of this journey came at the beginning, when Marty said to me, "We're not going to remove the tumor; now tell me why."

I remember I stumbled with some talk of the immune system, and he screamed into the phone, "*That's right!* We are going to keep his immune system on high alert, and he's going to live with it. We don't touch the tumor."

Now, understand that when a tumor is found, and a doctor tells you that he isn't touching it, my guess is that most people would be pissed off and think he was too lazy to do his job. Or he's too smart to do what's expected. Too instinctual to ignore the immune system's response to disease. Too insightful to walk us down the road that would surely lead to a life cut short. That precious life that I was desperate to extend, not only to save him, but my own sanity. The thought of losing the love of my life was too much to bear. Certainly not like this.

Cesar went on to be treated, month after month, with the highest level of care and focus. After the first few months, his tumor shrank by about 70 percent. Sometimes it was barely noticeable, and Cesar was thriving. Not acting like a sick dog at all, he had boundless energy. Until that day I went into the city . . .

My sister and brother-in-law were staying with me

during their summer vacation, and I had errands to run in downtown Manhattan. I was only gone for the day and returned before sundown to grim faces and weighted silence. I said to my family, "Where is Cesar?" They replied, "He's lying down, Maggie, he was falling over all day, and he can't get himself back up. He's really weak. It might be the end."

I remember feeling nothing. I walked right past them and said, "Let me see him." When I got to my boy, he was quite weak but stood for me anyway, albeit a little wobbly. I greeted him as enthusiastically as I always did, and he lit up. I felt no fear. I told everyone he was fine, and he was allowed to have weak moments. They replied that it wasn't a moment, it was all day. I didn't believe it, and neither did Cesar. We silently communicated our strength to each other while eyes darted across the room and elbows were nudged into one another's sides as if I didn't understand my own animal. By rights, they weren't wrong in their assessment. They just didn't know us, and they certainly didn't know Marty.

The weakness increased that night, and in the next five days he ran a fever so high his skin was burning in my hands. He couldn't move, he couldn't eat or drink. All he could do was allow me to encase him in ice packs and pray the fever would break. Meg and Marty brought all their daughters over, and we set up a mini-hospital in front of my bed. Meg taught me how to change his IV bag and give him rest from the drip when needed. I kept taking his temp on the hour and continued to talk him through what was now extremely clear to all of us.

Cesar was having a healing crisis.

Marty had warned me about this possibility. After the years of holistic treatment and pumping his body with all the "goods," it could all come to a head and he would have to fight for his life. If he made it out the other side, Marty and Meg told me, he would be fine until the end of his days. If he didn't, that was just going to be the cost of giving him an extra year of vibrant life instead of a slow and lethargic death. Then Marty also said, "If he *does* make it, don't be surprised if that tumor gets even smaller."

I never left my boy's side, and in my heart I had no fear. I told him, and myself, "This isn't the end." I told him his body was fighting for the other side, and as Marty said, it would be up to him. I told him I was ready for anything, but that in my heart I was certain he was coming back to me.

Then, on day five, the fever broke. Cesar stood. I cried the kind of tears that only faith brings. Faith in Marty, and his wisdom. Faith in Meg and her support. Faith in their girls for their unending compassion. Faith in the love and trust in the miracle of the method.

Cesar lived with cancer and his tumor still in his body—but even smaller after his crisis—for the next two and a half years. He enjoyed *vibrant* health, and our years together were the best years of his life with me. A German shepherd, he died at the age of sixteen. He never lived another sick day in his life; this was the definition of the long game—a vision for wellness that extends beyond the medical profession and into the spirit of who we are and what we value.

If you want to heal, you first have to believe in healing.

You must see it and live it in all that you do. This is who Marty is, and whom I have been blessed to know as not only my doctor, but as my family. The Goldsteins never gave up on my boy, and I am forever in their debt for giving me the gift of his life.

As Marty journeys forward into "retirement," his dreams and his family's dreams for him are finally coming true. I know that I have always seen him as leading the veterinary medical establishment in a different direction. One that will change the course of animal welfare forever. He will do it, and all I know is . . . I'm entirely blessed to witness it.

Watch out, world, here comes trouble! Love you, Marty!

Here is just how much I owe to Maggie in her support of my life and vision. Maggie became involved with this great product-development/educational/marketing company with the uniquely appropriate name the Golden Hippo. Her line is called ActivatedYou, and from the get-go I have been taking her probiotic, green-drink, plant-based omegas, and digestive-enzyme supplements daily.

Not too long ago, I reached the time in my life when I had to make the transition from staying in an examination or treatment room every day—getting to only several patients and educating a few people. I knew I could reach millions with this so-needed work, so I searched for options that would help me in this endeavor while being able to support my family and get my three daughters through college. Maggie kept telling me, "You need to hook up with the Hippo!"

Finally, after months of her convincing the "Head Hippo,"

Craig Clemens, that he needed to bring me on in addition to his twenty-six lines for humans to enter the arena of animal care, he agreed. We did a three-way conference call, and again, as they say, the rest is history. My Dr. Marty Pets line of freeze-dried raw diet and incredibly well-designed, high-quality supplements—based on my almost half a century of experience—are now available across the country. Combined with Golden Hippo's remarkable marketing skills to bring my education out to the masses, we have together created one of the great breakthroughs in my career and life.

It's one of the most rewarding things ever for me to hear how professional my presentations are regarded, but even more important are the testimonials streaming in thanking me for helping and even saving the lives of peoples' companions. I even get contacted by conventional veterinarians to discuss how their nonresponsive patients got better once they started administering one or several of my products.

And I now have a revenue stream that supports my life without my having to stay working patient by patient (again as indicated in the last line of my first book). Thank you, Maggie Q, for having the insight and then helping to make this happen. I am forever grateful we met.

THE AMAZING RODNEY HABIB AND PLANET PAWS

Now here's something I am extremely proud and elated to be part of—the story of Rodney Habib and Planet Paws. It goes something like this. Years ago, my receptionist told me that some guy named Rodney wanted to come to Smith Ridge on Friday to do a film interview with me. Whiskers—the incredible health food store for pets and great buddies of mine—was somehow involved. So, I called Whiskers and said that this Rodney guy must have me confused with my brother, but they said, "No, it's you." Believe me, I had no desire for this to happen.

Days later, my receptionist told me that this Rodney guy from Canada was on the phone. His flight got canceled, and he wanted to know if I would be willing to come in on Sunday to do the interview. Now I really had no desire for this interview to happen. As I explained to my receptionist how to nicely tell this guy to go away, I decided—mostly out of sheer curiosity—to call him myself to ask him who the heck he was, then politely tell him to scratch off. I'm fairly certain that he thought our interview was already established, but in my mind, there was no way—especially on my valuable Sundays off from working at my clinic.

So, as I was talking with Rodney—totally ignoring his plea for me to come in on an extremely rare and valuable weekend day off—he blurted out, "Do you like maple syrup?"

"What?" I asked him who set him up because harvesting my own maple syrup from my own maple trees and going through the extensive process of boiling it off—forty gallons of sap collected from the trees to make just one gallon of syrup—is a hobby more dear to me than any other.

Rodney replied, "No one. But if you let me come interview you, I will bring you bottles of the finest maple syrup in the world from Nova Scotia."

Without thinking twice, I immediately responded, "You're on! I'll meet you at my clinic Sunday morning!"

And the rest is history. Here's my dearest buddy, Rodney:

A SWEET GIFT

BY RODNEY HABIB

Founder, Planet Paws[1]

I remember when I got my first gig at *Dogs Naturally*, the number one dog magazine in the world. For my first assignment, they wanted me to write something about dog health. It was nerve-racking for me because here I was a first-time writer working for a magazine that was publishing articles by some of the world's greatest veterinarians, pro trainers, nutrition experts, and more. How on earth was I going to stand out from all these brilliant people and inspire readers?

Then it suddenly clicked—I knew what I was going to do.

I thought to myself, "I'm going to get on a plane, I'm going to fly to New York, and I'm going to sit down with Dr. Marty Goldstein for my first interview ever." The only problem was that I didn't know him, and he didn't know me. And here's a Canadian from Nova Scotia with no connections, though I was just starting to make some waves on the internet. I would fly to New York and leave it to the fate of the universe—I just felt deep inside that this guy would meet with me.

So, I called Smith Ridge and explained to the receptionist that I wanted to schedule an in-person interview with Dr. Marty so I could write my article for *Dogs Naturally*. She told me that Dr. Marty had an agent and that I would need to make arrangements through the agency.

"I just want you to leave one note," I said. "My name is Rodney Habib, I'm from Canada. I have a dog who was very sick and who changed my whole life. Dr. Marty's book was one of the first ones I picked up to get that information. I'm going to get on a plane and I'm going to fly down there. Just tell him I have nothing to give him—I have no money. I have nothing in my life that would be of value to him. But, being from Nova Scotia, one of the things that we do have is the very best maple syrup in the world. I'm going to bring Dr. Marty a vintage bottle of the most prized possession of my province." I had no idea that Marty was a huge fan of maple syrup, and I didn't know that this message was never relayed to Dr. Marty.

So I booked the flight and hoped for the best. I had to borrow money from my dad just to buy the ticket.

The day arrived to fly to New York—a Saturday. I checked my bags, got on the plane, and turned my phone to airplane mode as we taxied to the runway. While we were getting ready to take off, unbeknownst to me Marty had made plans to take his family skating for the weekend, which meant he wouldn't be available to do the interview. He called me to reschedule the interview that I thought was set up, but I later learned he had not only been un-aware of it but had no intention of doing it.

Just as Marty was punching my number into his phone to make the call, the airline captain announced that, be-cause of some debris on the runway, the plane would have to hold in place until it was cleared away. So, while we waited, I took my phone off airplane mode, and lo and behold, Marty's call came through.

I was crouched down in the back of the plane, talking with Dr. Marty. He told me that he had promised his family that he would take them skating for the weekend and for me not to get on the plane—we would have to re-schedule the interview that had never existed in the first place.

My plane was just a couple of minutes from lifting off, so I told him my whole story: "Look, here's the deal. I borrowed my father's savings to buy a plane ticket and I'm just about to take off. If you meet with me, you'll help me inspire a lot of people. I promise to make the best article and the best video that I can possibly make."

When that appeared to not be working, I said to him, "Do you like maple syrup?"

"What? How do you know that—did someone set you up?"

Boom—that was it. I didn't realize that harvesting and processing his own maple syrup was one of Dr. Marty's favorite pastimes. What do you know—he canceled going along on his family's skating trip for this young kid from Nova Scotia.

He was so gracious and said, "I don't know who you

are, but I can hear the fire in your belly, and I know you have a sick dog."

"If I lose my dog, I don't want her to die in vain. I want to be able to say that I did everything to inspire others on her behalf, and she would be that matchstick for me to achieve that goal."

Marty opened up his clinic on Sunday, and he sat down with me for the interview. My hands were shaking—I didn't know the questions to ask because I'm not a reporter. But Marty gave me the interview of a lifetime, and I was in awe that I was sitting across from this man.

After the interview, I returned home to Canada and wrote my heart out. The article made the front page of the magazine—they pushed me in front of everyone else—and things exploded for me after that.

I'm blessed the way that things have gone in my life and my career. Later on, I worked on some projects with Facebook, and they helped me build my first studio—the Creator's Lounge in Dartmouth, Nova Scotia—to channel content out to people. I wanted Marty to be my first interview, I wanted him to bless and christen my studio. I knew all the execs at Facebook would be watching that day. Just a few months before the interview, I was flown to Facebook headquarters, and Mark Zuckerberg invited me to speak onstage. Zuckerberg, Sheryl Sandberg, and a bunch of other people were there. They all wanted to know whom I was going to have on as my first guest.

"A veterinarian named Dr. Marty Goldstein," I told them.

Thank you, Dr. Marty.

Rodney's Planet Paws has become the largest pet-information site on the planet. Over a year ago, he sent me a Facebook stat: in a two-year period, he received more than 534 million page views—not just hits.

When I was at the AHVMA conference filming scenes for *The Dog Doc* more than four years ago, he took out his iPhone, put it on a tripod, hit a special black FB app given to him by one of the head people at Facebook, and did an impromptu interview with me in the lobby. In just seven minutes, we got 1.29 million views from all around the world.

I am so proud of Rodney and all he has accomplished, and I am pleased to have been an inspiration to him as he began his remarkable journey to properly educate millions of pet parents—bringing them the best and most current information, news, and knowledge about animal nutrition and health.

THE DOG DOC

BY CINDY MEEHL

Founder, Cedar Creek Productions[2]

I met Marty Goldstein twenty-nine years ago. I had a six-year-old shar-pei named Coco, who would randomly spike crazy-high fevers, go rigid, and be incapacitated. Her veterinarians had chronically put her on antibiotics and steroids. It became an endless cycle. At just six years of age, she was dying. My veterinarian told me she had never seen a shar-pei live past six, and she called the unexplained illness and high fevers "shar-pei syndrome." I was devastated! I left the clinic and went to a pet food store, where a woman noticed me crying and asked what was wrong. I told her that my dog was dying, and the vet couldn't save her.

This angel of a woman told me to go see Dr. Marty Goldstein. Quite skeptical that anyone could help, I called for an appointment and explained that Coco was in critical condition. That same evening, my phone rang at around 11:00 P.M. A cheery voice on the end of the line asked for me and told me he was Marty Goldstein. This was re-markable in itself because he didn't know me, and Coco wasn't even his patient (yet). He spent thirty minutes on the phone with me explaining how the body heals, and that with Coco we were chronically suppressing some-thing that was clearly trying to get out of the body. He explained everything in a commonsense way, and those thirty minutes resonated with me in the most profound way you could imagine. He took away my fear and dread of the high fevers and impending death. I felt we had a chance to save Coco, and that is exactly what we did!

What I witnessed over the next two months was noth-ing short of a miracle. We started by taking her off the an-tibiotics and steroids that she had been on for so long and began a program of supplements and homeopathics that allowed Coco to detox naturally. This was all she needed. This dog who had been acting as if she were old and feeble transformed back into a playful happy puppy! This spec-tacular transformation made me change the medical path for my whole family and rethink how we view health and medicine. Needless to say, I continued to take all my future dogs to him.

Fast-forward twenty-five years, and I felt passionate about sharing Dr. Marty and his clinic and philosophy with the world. We all want our pets to be with us as long as possible, and to live without pain and in good health. His way of thinking is so different and so much more effective that I want it to live forever. I believe that most people have lost sight of what true health is, and I would hope that they would find that vision in the same way I did.

We put together an incredible team of filmmakers and spent three years filming more than three hundred hours at the Smith Ridge clinic. I was hoping that a deep dive "behind the scenes" of the clinic would leave me still believing as strongly as I did in their methods, but I wanted to document what an integrative practice looked like. It exceeded my expectations!

So many people who came through their doors had stories as miraculous as mine, and they were so grateful to have a clinic that could offer something different and less invasive for their pets. I repeatedly heard how the energy was so different from that of any other vet clinic they had been to before, and their dogs were happy to be there, whereas they had been upset by other places.

I have to attribute that to the energy that Marty brought to that clinic. When he walks in the door, he is like a kid in a candy store. Always exuberant and cheerful, he lifts everyone's spirits, including his patients'. He taught me something so important about our feelings toward illness and disease and how we transmit those to our animals. When we focus on the disease and the doom and gloom of how it is manifesting, we project that energy to our sensitive pets. They are so in tune to us that our moods affect them. He is the master of bringing hope to any situation, and I believe it is something we all need to learn. It makes a huge difference. It is part of his magic that is so incredible and not often understood by many doctors for all species.

Marty Goldstein is a unique human being, and I am so glad that I captured that magic before he retired. We are doing an educational series from the three hundred hours of footage we filmed for the documentary, and I hope that veterinarians and pet parents alike will be able to learn a lot more about what this clinic has been about and how to make their pets live long and healthy lives. Marty is helping me put that together, and we hope it will be available soon after the film is released.

I am so honored to know him as a doctor and a friend along with his wife, Meg. I believe that God puts you in places where you should be and grow. I am positive he brought me into the world of Marty Goldstein and will be forever grateful that I have learned from the master!

THE WOMAN BEHIND THE MAN

We've all heard the saying "the woman behind the man." How many Academy Award winners of the male gender have professed to millions of television viewers that they could never have done it without the support of "my wife"?

Well, with me, it's the same.

Almost none of what I wanted to and did accomplish would have happened without my better half, Meg. As the 1990s were coming to a close, just after finishing my first book, one day I decided that I was done looking for Miss Right. I was convinced she didn't exist. Then, the very next day, a young lady interviewed for a job at Smith Ridge—she had come home from college for half a semester to recover from an illness and was looking for a job while she figured out what she wanted to do in life.

Meg was hired as a receptionist, and the rest is history. Her love for animals and what took place at the clinic made her decide not to go back to college. We dated, married, and had three incredible daughters in the coming years.

But even in our early days of dating, I noticed that my own dogs of many years instantly had an affinity for Meg that surpassed what they had for me. She worked in every department and section of the hospital—from receptionist, to technician, to running the supplement-ordering department, to running lab analyses, and much more. Right about the time we were married, my business was on the rocks financially, and it appeared that bankruptcy was the only solution. To me, opting for that would have been like giving up on a cancer patient. I hired an incredibly business-savvy manager, and over the years—with incredible work diligence—we turned it all around.

Meg was off having and raising our three daughters, and after a decade—as she was able to start coming back to work—we both sensed an inappropriate control issue involving the business manager, coupled with a disturbing crash in the business itself. Things could not be worked out, and my wife and I found ourselves with a nationally renowned veterinary clinic once again in financial distress, and neither of us had the knowledge to run a business that surpassed that of a senior in high school. But then I watched Meg—who had gained experience in every department—come in and take charge, and within one year Smith Ridge was in more stable condition than it had ever been. It was this alone that finally enabled me to sell a financially healthy clinic to one of my highly trained associates, Dr. Jenna, allowing me to change my personal trajectory while making sure that the foundational mission of Smith Ridge remained in place.

Here are a couple of nitty-gritty stories that exemplify how Meg and I worked together.

We had a patient named Kara, a beautiful black-and-white greyhound. She came down with a serious illness—initially believed to be the result of a foreign body in her intestines. Surgery didn't find anything conclusive. Then she went into a severe autoimmune crisis, and the only thing recommended by four doctors at a specialty facility in Connecticut was humane passage. Not accepting that, her pet parents brought Kara daily to Smith Ridge for intravenous vitamin C therapies.

Unfortunately, while Kara was undergoing the therapy, we were hit by one of the worst snowstorms ever, and the governor of Connecticut closed all the highways. What to do? Meg and I just took Kara home with us.

Meg was pregnant with our first daughter, Emma. Our home had the kitchen and the living room on the main floor, and bedrooms in the basement. Kara stayed sprawled out upstairs in the living room, unable to get up and on IV therapy most of the day. At 3:00 A.M., Meg awoke to hear, through the ceiling, that Kara had just urinated, so she went upstairs to clean up. I also awoke, and at that moment it hit me—that Kara's severe anemia, jaundice, and liver and kidney failure could be caused by a disease I personally had never before seen in my clinical career: leptospirosis.

What also hit me was that this disease, spread via urine, causes severe problems in human fetuses. "Oh my God!" I thought as I ran upstairs to get pregnant Meg away from the urine. Too late. Her job was done. The next morning, just four hours later, I called Kara's parents to tell them that I unfortunately had to get Kara out of our house. The snow was at least one and a half feet high with drifts up to five feet, and Kara's parents had to get special permission from the police to enter state roads, while I trucked through the snow on unplowed roads in my Jeep. Kara's parents transferred her home, and she went on to live a happy, healthy life for nine more years.

And then there was Cleatis, a Boston terrier. I start almost all my PowerPoint presentations with Cleatis, even professionally to veterinary groups and universities I have been invited to speak at. "Let's cut to the chase," I'll propose to the audience. "Cleatis is a powerful wake-up call to the tremendous benefits to patients of incorporating alternative therapies into conventional veterinary medicine." Here's his story.

Before the age of one, he was brought to me at the edge of shock—hemorrhaging from his rectum after more than $14,000 worth of medical therapy at a good veterinary specialty hospital near Smith Ridge. That was back in 2004, so imagine what that cost would be the equivalent of today. The four-page bill that resulted from his treatment showed the full extent of medical testing, diagnostics, and therapy that was performed—it was exhaustive. But the end result was a little pup almost in shock, dying.

I immediately gave him some homeopathic injections, got him on a low dose of intravenous vitamin C, stopped all conventional medications, and kept him in our clinic for a day, Friday into Saturday. I then sent him home on a home-cooked diet, a remedy, and just a few supplements. He responded well to the treatment—progressing from being an emaciated puppy with a swollen abdomen in terminal stages of starvation, into a robust, healthy dog who went on to lead a happy and healthy life for the next eight years. However, that all changed when Cleatis's pet parents called to tell us that he needed help—he was having trouble breathing.

Boston terriers are brachycephalic; that is, they are born with a pushed-in head that results in their characteristic flat nose and narrow airway. So, it's not out of the ordinary for these dogs to have trouble breathing. Added to that, Cleatis had a condition called elongated soft palate, and he had apnea. He had a harder time breathing with the soft long palate obstructing his airway.

We called in our favorite surgeon, Dr. Martin DeAngelis, to perform a soft palate resection—removing part of Cleatis's soft palate with a special laser surgical instrument. The surgery went well, but with all the swelling in the cramped space nature gave him, he could not breathe well—especially when he put his head down to try to sleep. My head technician, Kathy, was closely monitoring him through the night, and Cleatis was having big problems.

I got the call from Kathy, and Meg and I carted our three young daughters to the hospital at midnight to try to surgically implant a tube into Cleatis's trachea so he could breathe better and get some sleep. The procedure worked well enough, but Cleatis needed our close supervision nonstop. He made it through the following morning and afternoon, but then at around 1:00 A.M. I was again piling the family into our minivan to perform another surgery on Cleatis so he could breathe. Going into the weekend, we took Cleatis home with us, and with our family barely sleeping for two days in a row, it appeared all was safe. Meg said that, as a reward to the kids, I should take them to see one of the Disney princess movies that was showing at a local theater. Of course, being at the movies means cell phones off.

As fate would have it, Meg was with Cleatis in our backyard, and the breathing tube was working great. He positioned himself to poop, then all of a sudden, he started to fall backward—turning purple with his eyes rolled up into the back of his head. Meg ran over to him and picked him up—she saw that his trachea tube was caked with bloody mucus. She was tempted to pull out the trachea tube in hopes that Cleatis would be able to breathe, but she instead decided to just suck it out. So, she put her mouth on the tube and sucked the obstruction out of Cleatis's airway—saving his life. Eventually, Cleatis recovered, and we were rewarded with two good bottles of Opus One wine.

Meg is my best friend and partner in every way, and the

luckiest day of my life was when she applied for the receptionist job at Smith Ridge all those years ago.

COMFORT, CARE, AND LOVE

BY MEG GOLDSTEIN

I have loved animals for as long as I can remember. Working with animals was something I knew I was going to be doing for the rest of my life. Eventually, I concluded that I didn't just want to love them. I wanted to be their caregiver, their confidant, and their voice. I think in every human hospital they say nurses know more than doctors about patients. This is true in the vet field as well. Technicians are a vital part of the practice and know more about each patient and their emotional signs—pain, fear, love, anger, and more. This is what I wanted to be—I wanted to be the person who understood each patient and gave comfort, care, and love.

In the documentary *The Dog Doc,* there is a clip of me saying that what attracted me to Marty was that he made me laugh. This is true, but the most attractive quality he had then—and still has today—is his ethics and love for the animals. Practicing *physician do no harm* in every sense of the phrase is the true reason I am with him today. (Along with a few other reasons . . . LOL!)

Back in the 1990s, Marty was still under scrutiny for some of the methods he practiced—especially the utilization of natural remedies to sometimes reverse disease but most of all to give patients quality of life. Watching him convince pet parents with confidence and passion that he could help their beloved pets was something I hadn't seen with any vets I had previous experience with. Marty spent an hour or more with each patient and their pet parents—unraveling the knots of fear and hopelessness that conventional vets had instilled in them. That was probably when I first realized that he was passionate and different, and I admired that about him.

In the early days, we would hang out on the couch and watch football or watch a movie while Marty worked through a *huge* pile of patient files. Working up nutritional protocols for each patient, going through blood work from another vet hospital, making follow-up phone calls, and lots more. Yup, we spent a lot of time on that ugly green couch. He would stay up till 3:00 to 4:00 A.M., get a few hours of sleep, and start the day all over again bright and early. For me, the best part was I got to hang out with Clayton (miniature poodle), Nina (Pomeranian), Jasmine (Siamese), and Geter (domestic long hair).

We took many, many sick patients home instead of transferring them to twenty-four-hour emergency hospitals. I fell in love with every single one of them. Bringing patients home is not an easy task. They need to be monitored through the night, taken out to pee and poop every two or three hours because they are on IV, have IVs checked, have food prepared, and so on. Marty and I worked well together on those nights. We never questioned each other for bringing a sick patient home. Sometimes it was my idea to bring the patient home and sometimes it was Marty's. We worked together as a team to accomplish what was best for the patient. We knew every one of these patients missed their pet parents and their home. So, it was important for us to create the next best thing. Most of them did well away from home.

We had no sadness when we treated these patients. We worked to keep it positive and not come from negative/sympathetic emotions. The patients can tell when you get emotionally involved. I always felt that, as their caregiver, my place was to do everything I could to keep the patients comfortable and get them well so they could get home to be spoiled. I think almost all the patients who stayed with us did well because we didn't let our emotions burden their healing process. I knew when to let them be and when to push them.

We continued to bring patients home after we were married and had three young kids. Our daughters grew up with so many patients coming in and out of our lives, as well as our own four dogs and two cats. I believe that our daughters are caring, loving, and compassionate humans because of these experiences. I love that we have created this life together for our family where if any member feels an animal needs help or a home, we don't question or argue. We support one another's choices and bring them home.

We have created a lifestyle as a family to give every animal a chance at happiness. That gives us tremendous joy and satisfaction. We will continue to do what we can.

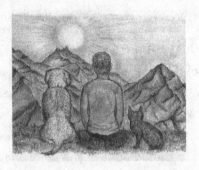

11

LOOKING TO THE FUTURE

Where Do We Go from Here?

The reasonable man adapts himself to the world;
the unreasonable one persists in trying to
adapt the world to himself.
Therefore, all progress depends on the unreasonable man.
—GEORGE BERNARD SHAW

I have used these words written by George Bernard Shaw—
one of my favorite quotes of all time—to open almost every
seminar I have given over the past thirty years. It's a constant
reminder why it's okay for me to sometimes seem so unreasonable to many in my chosen profession. But I have also
been gratified to see so many veterinarians adopt the "radical" treatments that I have championed for so long. There is
a light at the end of this very long tunnel.

In the first chapter of this book, I told the story about

how I was invited back to speak at my alma mater Cornell on a subject now so vital for the new generation of veterinary students to embrace: integrative veterinary medicine. Fortunately, my entire presentation—along with the Q&A afterward—was captured on film, and segments of it became the conclusion of my documentary, *The Dog Doc*.

A freshman, at Cornell for only three weeks, approached me after my talk. She wanted to share with me how moved she was by being exposed to this new way of thinking so early in her formal education. At that moment I realized that my seemingly unreachable life's dream might finally come to pass. As I mentioned in the first chapter, years before, Cornell's administration had surveyed the student body of the College of Veterinary Medicine. The survey revealed that 93 percent of students had an interest in alternative forms of therapy, but the wall of resistance I faced for decades ensured that these therapies did not become a part of the program.

But, has that wall finally begun to crumble? Have the resisters I've encountered along the way moved on—by retirement or even death? Was the way now clear for alternative treatments and protocols to enter the mainstream?

I learned conventional veterinary medicine well, and over my long career not only did I properly apply it to treat companion animals, but I also kept up as the profession evolved. Fortunately, I was also one of the earliest and foremost to delve into these more natural, biological therapies—some having been practiced for thousands of years. Integrating these approaches into everyday practice was as commonsense to me as $2 + 2 = 4$. But almost no one else saw that. Only the truth of the matter kept me alive from all the arrows that pierced my back.

Today, things are much different. At least seventeen of the thirty-one AVMA-accredited veterinary schools in the United States (54 percent) have veterinarians certified in or with an interest in acupuncture as faculty members or offer acupuncture to their clients through referral.[1]

Yes, of all the alternative therapies currently available, acupuncture is still the gateway for veterinarians to begin embracing these health modalities.

I find it funny now when I go to continuing-education seminars how, over and over, I hear my associates—many of whom used to criticize me—say, "You were so ahead of your time."

My answer to them is "What? Acupuncture has been around for thousands of years. I was just thirty-five years less behind than you!"

Now we have another aspect of this trend to discuss, and that is society's view of health care, even for companion animals. As I said to the students at Cornell, "The bandwagon is traveling in this direction. So, you need to make the choice to jump on now or eventually just be behind the times."

In chapter 5, we discussed Dr. Google and how it can cause more harm than good in the hands of well-meaning pet parents. One big problem I've seen is the censorship of alternative-medicine websites. Without going too far down this particular rabbit hole, I just want you to know that this has been an issue in the past, and I expect it to continue to be an issue in the future. As we go forward, this element that is so anti what I represented still exists—including the large social media sites that feel they have to censor alternative content and warnings about vaccines. The major drug companies have tremendous influence on our society and what we are allowed to read, what we are encouraged to consume, and the information that is allowed to make its way into our brains. Caveat emptor.

However, the vast knowledge on the internet also has an upside. I have heard it said that Google alone has increased the IQ of the human race up to a hundred points. Just think, almost anything you want to know is at your fingertips. This has tremendously raised the knowledge of veterinarians' clients. When their pet is ill, or when they want to know more about animal health care and wellness, they can take time and focus on research—often much more time and focus than the busy veterinarian whose schedule is jam-packed with patients.

A certain amount of ego attaches to doctors, who, through the intensive education to obtain their degrees, feel that they know best what's good for your animal companion. How could anyone who hasn't had the same education possibly know more than he or she does? What gives people the right to question the judgment of a licensed veterinarian?

From being the second, third, or even fourth opinion on thousands of cases, I have seen countless times how this has led to conflict when clients questioned their veterinarian on things they know to be correct. Unfortunately, it's often the veterinarian who has not been aware of the benefits of certain nutraceuticals or who has been educated to think that feeding a biologically appropriate diet to pets is not scientifically grounded.

Just by being open to the influx of new information and not allowing my ego to get in the way, I have learned so many things over the years from my clients and have passed it on to my associates. I use this knowledge to benefit my patients.

Over several decades, I have accumulated an impressive collection of animal pins, well up into the hundreds. A scene in *The Dog Doc* shows this collection, and not a day goes by that I am not wearing at least one distinctive pin. The forerunner of this pin collection, which dates back to my student days at Cornell—both undergraduate and while in vet school—was a collection of buttons with all sorts of thought-provoking or funny sayings and images. Large, small, rainbowed, psychedelic; I had many.

But one button in particular guided my life. I wore this small, simple button almost every day. Printed on the button was QUESTION AUTHORITY.

I still have that button, and more important, I still embrace its message. It's a message I want to pass on to you: When you feel fairly certain about a topic or situation concerning your animal companion's health and that opinion conflicts with your veterinarian's, stand your ground. Do not be rude or not listen to or respect the veterinarian's advice from many years of training and experience. But if something doesn't feel right, don't just give in.

I can't begin to tell you how many times my associates and I have reviewed patients' histories and learned that these dogs and cats were given their vaccinations due by calendar while being treated for illness. Their human parents first questioned this but then gave in—feeling sick themselves for allowing the shots to be administered, only leading to a worsening of the condition. And this is because their veterinarian—the university-trained expert with years of experience—decided not to question authority.

As I sit here writing the final chapter of this book, our race and planet are caught up in the COVID-19 pandemic. Thankfully our companion animals are not affected, but the point to make remains the same. Deep into the pandemic, there is no reported treatment except for the possibility of an old antimalarial drug and a few other medications. We just don't know yet.

Vaccination research is on a major push, but who knows what negative effects will result years from now from creating a vaccine and vaccinating the population on a fast track with hardly any clinical trials. But I am receiving information on things that *do* have beneficial effects in preventing and even helping to successfully treat affected patients. These things include liposomal vitamin C, oil of thyme, glutathione, black seed oil, and more.

But of all the reports I have both received and researched, the one thing that stands out to me is the potential benefit offered by vitamin C for both preventing and treating this virus—orally and especially by intravenous administration. This is the same therapy I used more than forty years ago to successfully treat cases of the viral diseases distemper and parvovirus that appeared to be terminal or hopeless. I am particularly intrigued by a report published by the Shanghai Medical Association claiming IV vitamin C therapy is beneficial against COVID-19. Keep in mind, China is where this disease arose.

Even more significant are the results of vitamin C infusion for the treatment of coronavirus-infected pneumonia, reported by the National Institutes of Health's National Library of Medicine. Here are two direct quotes from the research report:

"Early clinical studies have shown that vitamin C can effectively prevent this process."

"Therefore, during the current epidemic of SARI [referring to COVID-19)], it is necessary to study the clinical efficacy and safety of vitamin C for viral pneumonia through randomized controlled trials."[2]

With this coming from the highest level of our federal government—and also being studied, used, and reported in foreign countries—then why is this not even mentioned in the current daily press conferences by the president of this country, his cabinet, or staff as *even a potential treatment* when currently there are no others?

Low and behold, a report just hit the *New York Post* regarding hospitals in New York City that are successfully using IV vitamin C therapy to treat COVID-19.[3] Unfortunately, the doses presented in the article are way lower than those we have been using for decades in our animal patients and those I have studied that are being used to treat humans. But at least it's a start.

I recently attended three screenings of *The Dog Doc* at the Boulder International Film Festival, and I was gratified that the film was so well embraced by the more than five hundred people who watched it. The last screening was in the beautiful First United Methodist Church, built of native stone in 1892. It was awe-inspiring to the point that, during my introduction of the film, I asked attendees to consider this question: "And what is *God* spelled backwards?"

But something else happened at the festival that made a lasting impression on me—summing up my life's work. One of the featured films was Robbie Robertson's *Once Were Brothers*. Robbie, who wrote a majority of the songs for the rock group The Band, spoke after the screening. He shared that, in 1966, when the group—then known as The Hawks—toured Australia and Europe with Bob Dylan, they received only boos and items tossed at them from the audiences. Why? Because Dylan's fans were incensed that he had added an electric rock 'n' roll set to his regular acoustic-guitar, folk-music concert repertoire. However, they continued their tour undaunted because, as Robbie explained, "We were on a mission. The rest of the world didn't get it. They just needed to catch up."

While there is still some way to go, I am pleased that the rest of the world is finally catching up to the benefits of integrative veterinary practice. They get it.

So here we have a major focus for my own future. I have completed almost a half century of clinical work as an integrative veterinarian, gathering a large quantity of case documentation and experience. Once again, as my last book concluded, "The challenge seems overwhelming sometimes, but we have to keep at it. Dog by dog, cat by cat. One animal at a time."

Now, more than two decades later, we have the future laid out in front of us. But what kind of future will it be? I can tell you one thing for sure—it's going to be quite different from the future most of us imagined. I am committing every fiber in my being to drive forward—through this book, the documentary film, my product and educational company, and other media—and serve as a spokesperson for whatever benefits the health and welfare of our companion animals and society as a whole.

The knowledge and the data are here, and available. We just need to get it *there*. Where it works for all.

The times of one animal at a time are gone. Now, through *The Spirit of Animal Healing*, it's time to Save Our Favorite Kingdom!

ACKNOWLEDGMENTS

No man is an island. No man can do something such as this alone. The support system I have had behind writing this book has been huge and long-standing. My deep and sincere and everlasting thanks to each and every one of you who has loved and supported me throughout my career and life. I am the luckiest man alive.

To my wife, Meg: For your support, wisdom, and love. Without it, *none* of this could ever have happened.

To my three beautiful daughters, Emma, Hana, and Ayla: You remind me every day that my life was finally complete and all about this wonderful bond we have with our animal companions. And a special thanks to Emma and Ayla for your remarkable artwork for each chapter header, depicting some of the family companions we shared our lives with over the years . . . and their ancestors.

To Peter Economy, my cowriter: For making this process so effortless and enjoyable, and with your skills and contributions—a work way beyond my expectations.

To Jim Moscowitz, my adviser, my CFO, my confidant, and my dearest friend: Life finally started to work when you came on board. And to your incredible wife, Tina Redecha: Without you, none of what I wrote about Jim could have happened—LOL.

To Daniela Rapp and Giles Anderson, my editor at St. Martin's and literary agent respectively: You made this process so supportive and easy for me to accomplish.

To *all* the contributors: Cindy Meehl; Rodney Habib; Dr. Jean Dodds; Meg Goldstein; Robert F. Kennedy Jr.; Dr. Rick Palmquist; Dr. Ian Billinghurst; Dr. Ron Schultz; Dr. Jacqueline Ruskin; Dr. Andrew Wakefield; Pat, Deborah, and Alane Ziemer; Jeffrey Smith; Dr. Rob Silver; Dr. George Zabrecky; Dr. Karen Becker; Dr. Margo Roman; Dr. David Lerner; Sonya Fitzpatrick and Emma Kiper; Dr. Martin DeAngelis; Larry and Lana Canova; John Hendrickson; Steve Sayegh and Elsa; Lance Fargo and Blitz; Wendy Coren; and Dave Lundquist. Your contributions elevated this book and my life to a much higher plateau, and I am eternally grateful. My respect to each of you—your work and support go far beyond the scope of this book.

And, in no particular order, to *all* those who mean so much: Helmut and Patricia Meissner; Bob, Susan, Abbey, and Merritt Goldstein; Aunt Selma, Joni Evans; Mary and Barry Curtis; Andrew Loog Oldham; Eileen Cohhn; Maureen Hamill; Andrea Eastman; Annie Schulhof; Beverly Carter and Bill Pickens; Phil and Randi Klein; Grant Aleksander and Sherry Ramsey; Barbara Lazaroff; Carol Alt; Marisa Tomei; Keith and Hayley Carradine; Gary Epstein; the Rudin family; Frank Cardaci; Steve Rosdal; Michael and Claudia Franks; Julia Henriques, Gregg Oehler, Tim Hockley and Dana Cox; Dick Button and Dennis Grimaldi; Ed Burns and Christy Turlington; Chevy and Jayni Chase; Jeff Kurtz; Jocelyn Santos; Jordan Rubin; Ty and Charlene

Bollinger; Steven Klein; Tom and Karen Lewandowski; Ursula and Rob Covino; Mike and Suzi Covino; Grandma and Papa; Dr. Greg Ogilvie, Dr. Mark Nesselson, and Dr. Bob Harmon; Dana Scott; Julia Henriques, Gregg Oehler, Tim Hockley and Dana Cox, Frank Pompilio; Stormy Farley; Maria Echevarria; Roger Goodman; Tamar Geller; Dr. Rick Joseph; Dr. John Parks; Beth Pratt; Ingrid Newkirk; Dr. Maggie Coffey; Lloyd and Maddie Kushner; Sharon and Mike Quisenberry; Ruth Vitale; Dr. Greg Ogilvie, Dr. Mark Nesselson, Dr. Bob Harmon, and anyone I might have missed. I am eternally grateful to each of you and am fortunate to have you in my life. Thank you from the bottom of my heart.

To Smith Ridge: Thank you for being my vehicle all these years, and thank you to Dr. Jenna and all the staff for continuing my work forward.

To Cindy Meehl: Not only for having the vision and wherewithal with your amazing Cedar Creek Productions staff to create *The Dog Doc*, but also for the tremendous support you have given me over the last thirty years.

To Rodney Habib: To be able to take the vision of a Sunday interview, and through your creation of Planet Paws, turn it into the largest animal-wellness educational engine on this planet.

To Maggie Q: For your amazing humanitarian work for the animals, and also for creating my position at Golden Hippo, which enabled me to accomplish my dreams in my lifetime. And, most important, for being you, as my friend.

To Craig Clemens, founder of Golden Hippo: Thank you for having the vision for creating the Dr. Marty Pets line, and to Aaron Channon, Tim Neumann, and the whole Dr. Marty Pets team for these incredible products and education helping me truly impact the health of millions of our four-legged family members globally.

To Martha Stewart and Oprah Winfrey: For accepting my work into your lives and helping me spread the word on the remarkable platforms you created.

To Squeeki, Cesar, Daniel, Cleatis, Blitz, Ocean, Sofie, Kara, Edel, Nina, Clayton, Jasmine, Geter, and Taylor. Also to Kooper, Tilly, Joey, Redford, Tara, Sprout, Miko, Topi, Zots, Paco, Pickles, Blossom, Spotty, the horses Famous and Harvey, our bunny Porkchop, our rats Fiona and Remy and Ducky, Dove, and all the Chickens.

To the animals: We as a race need to love, cherish, respect, care for, honor, and, especially, learn from you.

Whatever goes upon four legs, or has wings, is a friend.
—*ANIMAL FARM*, GEORGE ORWELL

NOTES

INTRODUCTION: WHAT'S NEW?

1. https://www.dailydogstuff.com/us-pet-ownership-statistics/.
2. https://www.americanpetproducts.org/press_industrytrends
.asp.

1. HOW FAR HAVE WE COME?

1. Jalandris, *The Hall of Records, Second Edition* (Holistic Life
Travels, 1980), 7.
2. https://penntoday.upenn.edu/news/compound-derived
-mushroom-lengthens-survival-time-dogs-cancer-penn-vet
-study-finds.

3. INSIDE YOUR PET'S MIND AND BODY

1. https://education.seattlepi.com/animals-share-human-dna
-sequences-6693.html.
2. https://sciencing.com/animals-share-human-dna-sequences
-8628167.html.
3. https://www.science20.com/news_articles/juramaia_sinensis
_160millionyearold_fossil_pushes_back_mammal_evolution
-81971.
4. https://www.vox.com/the-goods/2019/8/12/20799061/pet
-supplement-industry-vitamins-dogs-cats.

5. https://www.avma.org/News/JAVMANews/Pages/170115a.aspx.

6. https://www.ncbi.nlm.nih.gov/pubmed/22121108.

7. https://well.blogs.nytimes.com/2011/08/03/calculating-the-real-age-of-your-dog/.

8. https://pets.webmd.com/dogs/how-to-calculate-your-dogs-age.

9. https://ntrs.nasa.gov/archive/nasa/casi.ntrs.nasa.gov/20030075722.pdf.

10. https://www.ncbi.nlm.nih.gov/pmc/articles/PMC3267855/; https://www.sciencedaily.com/releases/2019/02/190214093359.htm.

4. FOOD IS STILL WHERE IT STARTS

1. Martin Goldstein, DVM, *The Nature of Animal Healing* (Ballantine Books, 1999), 61.

2. https://www.nytimes.com/2014/08/03/magazine/who-made-that-dog-biscuit.html.

3. https://commons.wikimedia.org/wiki/File:1876_ad_for_Spratt%27s_Patent_Meat_Fibrine_Dog_Cakes.jpg.

4. http://news.bbc.co.uk/2/hi/asia-pacific/7843972.stm.

5. https://www.fda.gov/animal-veterinary/recalls-withdrawals/melamine-pet-food-recall-frequently-asked-questions.

6. https://www.accessdata.fda.gov/scripts/cdrh/cfdocs/cfCFR/CFRSearch.cfm?CFRPart=570&showFR=1.

7. https://www.aafco.org/Consumers/What-is-in-Pet-Food.

8. Code of Federal Regulations, Title 21, chap. 1, subchap. E, pt. 582.

9. Ibid., pt. 589.

10. https://talkspetfood.aafco.org/roleofaafco.

11. https://talkspetfood.aafco.org/readinglabels.

12. https://www.pfma.org.uk/types-of-dog-food.

13. https://www.dogsnaturallymagazine.com/why-aafco-guide lines-are-useless-for-raw-dog-food/.

14. Dr. Ian Billinghurst, *Food "Allergies" and Dr. B's BARF*, 4, https://www.academia.edu/8850065/Allergies_and_Dr._Bs_BARF.

15. https://drianbillinghurst.com/barf/.

16. https://healthypets.mercola.com/sites/healthypets/archive /2018/10/20/pet-food-extrusion.aspx.

17. https://www.fda.gov/animal-veterinary/outbreaks-and -advisories/fda-investigation-potential-link-between-certain -diets-and-canine-dilated-cardiomyopathy.

18. https://www.gmoseralini.org/roundup-toxic-heart-new-study/.

19. Natália Kovalkovičová and Irena Šutiaková, "Some Food Toxic for Pets," *Interdisciplinary Toxicology* 2 (3) (September 2009): 169–76.

20. Ibid.

21. Ibid.

22. Ibid.

23. https://www.cdc.gov/training/SIC_CaseStudy/Infection _Salmonella_ptversion.pdf.

24. https://www.cdc.gov/salmonella/pet-treats-07-19/index.html.

25. https://www.merckvetmanual.com/digestive-system/salmon ellosis/overview-of-salmonellosis.

5. THE TREMENDOUS POWER OF NUTRACEUTICALS

1. https://www.nytimes.com/1992/08/09/us/fda-steps-up-effort -to-control-vitamin-claims.html.

2. https://www.avma.org/News/JAVMANews/Pages/170115a .aspx.

3. https://health.gov/dietsupp/ch1.htm.

4. https://www.fda.gov/animal-veterinary/animal-food-feeds /product-regulation.

5. https://health.gov/dietsupp/ch1.htm.

6. https://talkspetfood.aafco.org/supplements.

7. http://www.fao.org/news/story/en/item/357059/icode/.

8. https://www.theglobeandmail.com/life/todays-fruits-vegetables -lack-yesterdays-nutrition/article4137315/.

9. Bernard Jensen, *Food Healing for Man* (Bernard Jensen, 1983), 41.

10. Shari Lieberman, Ph.D., and Ken Babal, C.N., *Maitake Mushroom and D-Fraction* (Woodland Publishing, 2004).

11. https://www.ncbi.nlm.nih.gov/pmc/articles/PMC6044372/.

12. https://penntoday.upenn.edu/news/compound-derived -mushroom-lengthens-survival-time-dogs-cancer-penn-vet -study-finds.

13. Ibid.

14. https://ww5.komen.org/BreastCancer/Aloe.html.

15. https://www.dogsnaturallymagazine.com/the-health-benefits -of-coconut-oil/.

16. https://www.ncbi.nlm.nih.gov/pmc/articles/PMC4681158/.

17. https://www.webmd.com/vitamins/ai/ingredientmono-993 /fish-oil.

18. https://www.who.int/malaria/media/artemisinin_resistance _qa/en/.

19. https://humanclinicals.org/champex.

6. OTHER REMARKABLE THERAPIES

1. https://www.ncbi.nlm.nih.gov/pubmed/23026007.

2. https://www.ncbi.nlm.nih.gov/pmc/articles/PMC3104015/.

3. https://www.ncbi.nlm.nih.gov/pmc/articles/PMC431183/.

4. https://riordanclinic.org/wp-content/uploads/2018/06/7a -PART-2-The-Riordan-IVC-Protocol_c.pdf.

5. https://siteman.wustl.edu/ncipdq/cdr0000742253/.

6. https://www.fda.gov/animal-veterinary/development-approval

-process/veterinary-regenerative-medicine-animal-cell-based-products.

7. https://vetstem.com/pdfs/6110-0007-002%20Quality%20of%20Life%20Handout.pdf.

8. https://vetstem.com/pdfs/Osteoarthritis%20and%20the%20Older%20Dog.pdf.

9. http://medivetbiologics.com/home/pet-owners/why-stem-cell-therapy/.

10. https://cfpub.epa.gov/npstbx/files/cwc_petwastefactsheet.pdf.

11. https://www.whole-dog-journal.com/health/digestion/fecal-transplants-for-dogs/.

12. https://www.purinainstitute.com/science-of-nutrition/promoting-gastrointestinal-health/gut-brain-axis.

13. https://www.dogsnaturallymagazine.com/dysbiosis-in-dogs-causes/.

14. Ibid.

15. http://www.mashvet.com/fecal-transplants.html.

16. https://mercola.fileburst.com/PDF/HealthyPets/Interview-DrMargoRoman-MicrobiomeRestorativeTherapy.pdf.

17. Ibid.

18. Ibid.

19. https://www.mskcc.org/trending-topics/fecal-transplants-proven-restore-health-promoting-bacteria-01.

20. E. Hartshorne, "On the Causes and Treatment of Pseudo-arthrosis and Especially That Form of It Sometimes Called Supernumerary Joint," *American Journal of Medecine* 1 (1841): 121–56.

21. https://www.businessinsider.com/steve-jobs-bill-gates-kids-compete-florida-horse-playground-2018-3#still-its-clear-that-many-of-the-vendors-peddling-goods-at-wellington-are-targeting-an-elite-set-of-riders-who-have-thousands-of-dollars-to-spend-on-things-such-as-horses-fly-bonnets-13.

22. http://ic.instantcustomer.com/go/80990/lead-page-3081.

23. https://www.magnawavepemf.com.

24. https://www.cancer.gov/about-cancer/treatment/types/surgery /hyperthermia-fact-sheet.

25. Ibid.

26. Ibid.

27. https://journals.plos.org/plosone/article?id=10.1371/journal .pone.0055937.

7. THE CURRENT STATE OF DOG AND CAT DISEASE

1. https://www.schoolofhealth.com/naturopathy/a-z-of -naturopathy/.

2. https://www.dailydogstuff.com/us-pet-ownership-statistics/.

3. https://www.americanpetproducts.org/press_industrytrends .asp.

4. https://www.instituteofcaninebiology.org/blog/do-dogs-have -more-cancer-than-other-mammals.

5. https://grca.org/wp-content/uploads/2015/08/cancergoldens .pdf.

6. https://www.sciencedirect.com/science/article/abs/pii/S109 6286798800078.

7. For more information, please visit www.drianbillinghurst.com.

8. https://holisticdentist.com.

9. https://www.aafa.org/allergy-facts/.

10. https://www.ahvma.org/wp-content/uploads/AHVMA-2017 -V46-Vaccinosis.pdf.

11. O. L. Frick and D. L. Brooks, "Immunoglobulin E Antibodies to Pollens Augmented in Dogs by Virus Vaccines," *American Journal of Veterinary Research* 44 (3) March 1983: 440–45 PMID: 6301317.

12. https://onlinelibrary.wiley.com/doi/10.1111/j.1600-065X .1978.tb01461.x.

13. https://www.purdue.edu/vet/cpb/files/documents/scott
-moncrieff_et_al-2006-journal_of_veterinary_internal
_medicine.pdf.

14. https://journals.sagepub.com/doi/10.1016/j.jfms.2006.03
.003.

15. https://bmcvetres.biomedcentral.com/articles/10.1186/s12917
-016-0633-8.

16. https://www.hemopet.org/dog-aberrant-behavior-thyroid
-dysfunction/.

17. http://www.coastalpoint.com/37113/feature/local-dog-has
-his-day-thanks-holistic-vet.

18. https://well.blogs.nytimes.com/2007/10/22/when-doctors
-steal-hope/.

8. DOCTOR, DO NO HARM

1. https://www.ncbi.nlm.nih.gov/pubmed/6301317.

2. https://www.ncbi.nlm.nih.gov/pubmed/28960714.

3. https://www.cdc.gov/vaccines/hcp/vis/vis-statements/mmr
.html.

4. https://calmatters.org/health/2019/09/california-new-law
-vaccination-medical-exemption/.

5. https://childrenshealthdefense.org/news/ca-sb-276-sb-714
-signed-into-law-by-gov-newsom/.

6. http://www.coastalpoint.com/47730/feature/maggie-s
-vaccine-protection-act-passed-legislature.

7. Ronald D. Schultz, "Duration of Immunity for Canine and Feline Vaccines: A Review," *Veterinary Microbiology* 117 (2006):
75–79.

8. W. J. Dodds, "Commentary: Vaccine Issues Revisited," *Advances in Vaccines & Vaccination Research*, in press; W. J. Dodds,
"Vaccine Issues and the World Small Animal Veterinary Association (WSAVA) Guidelines (2015–2017)," *Israel Journal of
Veterinary Medicine* 73 (2) (2018): 3–10.

9. https://www.whitehouse.gov/briefings-statements/remarks
-president-trump-vice-president-pence-members-coronavirus
-task-force-press-briefing-12/.

9. WALKING THROUGH YOUR PET'S SPIRITUAL WORLD

1. http://www.naturalhistorymag.com/universe/201367/cosmic
-perspective?page=2.
2. https://www.washingtonpost.com/science/2019/09/25/what
-makes-dogs-so-special-successful-love/.
3. https://www.mnn.com/family/pets/stories/6-medical-conditions
-that-dogs-can-sniff.
4. https://plan.core-apps.com/eb2019/abstract/75baa294-b5aa
-489c-8c74-d36144aca3c5.
5. https://www.nytimes.com/1981/10/06/science/ions-created
-by-winds-may-prompt-changes-in-emotional-states.html.
6. https://www.jems.com/2018/07/25/it-s-a-full-moon-tonight/.
7. https://www.usgs.gov/special-topic/water-science-school
/science/water-you-water-and-human-body?qt-science_center
_objects=0#qt-science_center_objects.
8. https://www.smithsonianmag.com/smithsonian-institution
/why-ancient-egyptians-loved-their-kitties-180965155/.
9. Pat Rodegast and Judith Stanton, *Emmanuel's Book II: The Choice for Love* (Bantam Books, 1989), 144.

10. TAILS BEYOND THE CLINIC

1. https://www.planetpaws.ca.
2. https://cedarcreekmedia.com/.

11. LOOKING TO THE FUTURE—WHERE DO WE GO FROM HERE?

1. http://people.tamu.edu/~e-tebeaux/ode/techwrite/Validity%20 of%20Acupuncture.pdf.
2. https://clinicaltrials.gov/ct2/show/NCT04264533.
3. https://nypost.com/2020/03/24/new-york-hospitals-treating -coronavirus-patients-with-vitamin-c/.

INDEX

ABOUT THE AUTHOR

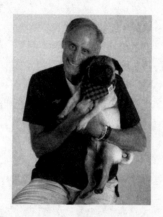

Dr. Marty Goldstein's Smith Ridge Veterinary Center is in South Salem, New York. He received his D.V.M. from the Cornell University College of Veterinary Medicine and has been at the forefront of integrative medicine for pets for decades. He has many cats and dogs, as well as a bunny, rats, birds, horses, and chickens, who all live to be old and healthy. Dr. Goldstein is also the author of *The Nature of Animal Healing*.